I1039265

Facilitating Learning in Healthcare

Health Sciences Library /
Bibliothèque des sciences de la santé
Hôpital régional de Sudbury Regional Hospital
41 chemin Ramsey Lake Road
Sudbury, ON P3E 5J1

ULLA Pharmacy Series

Editor in Chief

Prof Anthony C Moffat

The School of Pharmacy, University of London, UK

Members of the Editorial Advisory Board

Prof Patrick Augustijns, Katholieke Universiteit Leuven, Laboratory for Pharmacotechnology and Biopharmacy, Belgium

Prof Franco Bernini, University of Parma, Dipartimento di Scienze Farmacologiche, Biologiche e Chimiche Applicate, Italy

Prof Meindert Danhof, LACDR, Director of Research, the Netherlands

Prof Lennart Dencker, Uppsala University, Faculty of Pharmacy, Department of Pharmaceutical Biosciences, Sweden

Prof Elias Fattal, University Paris-South, Faculty of Pharmacy, France

Prof Sven Frokjaer, University of Copenhagen, Faculty of Pharmaceutical Sciences, Denmark

Prof Flemming Jorgensen, University of Copenhagen, Faculty of Pharmaceutical Sciences, Department of Medicinal Chemistry, Denmark

Prof Denis Labarre, University Paris-South, Faculty of Pharmacy, France

Prof Fred Nyberg, University Paris-South, Faculty of Pharmacy, France

Prof Patrizia Santi, University of Parma, Dipartimento Farmaceutico, Italy

Prof Nico Vermeulen, LACDR-Section of Molecular Toxicology, Department of Chemistry and Pharmacochemistry, the Netherlands

Other titles in the ULLA pharmacy series include:

Facilitating Learning in Healthcare

Edited by
Sarah Carter PhD
Research Manager, University of London School of Pharmacy, UK

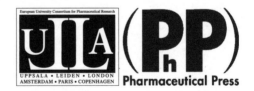

European University Consortium for Pharmaceutical Research

UPPSALA • LEIDEN • LONDON
AMSTERDAM • PARIS • COPENHAGEN

Pharmaceutical Press

Published by Pharmaceutical Press

1 Lambeth High Street, London SE1 7JN, UK

© Royal Pharmaceutical Society of Great Britain 2012

(**PP**) is a trade mark of Pharmaceutical Press
Pharmaceutical Press is the publishing division of the
Royal Pharmaceutical Society

First published 2012

Typeset by River Valley Technologies, India
Printed in Great Britain by T J International, Padstow, UK

ISBN 978 0 85369 954 5

All rights reserved. No part of this publication may be reproduced,
stored in a retrieval system, or transmitted in any form or by any means,
without the prior written permission of the copyright holder.
   The publisher makes no representation, express or implied,
with regard to the accuracy of the information contained in this book
and cannot accept any legal responsibility or liability for any errors or
omissions that may be made.
   The right of Sarah Carter to be identified as the author of this
work has been asserted by her in accordance with the Copyright,
Designs and Patents Act, 1988

A catalogue record for this book is available from the British Library.

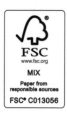

FSC
www.fsc.org
MIX
Paper from
responsible sources
FSC® C013056

Contents

Preface

This book was written because increasingly people from non-teaching backgrounds are asked to teach undergraduate or postgraduate healthcare students and practitioners. Not only do they have little or no teaching experience, but they have very little time in which to learn how to teach effectively. This book is a quick practical guide for these individuals. Although its authors are predominantly from a pharmacy background, the content is applicable for teachers from any background – healthcare practitioners, postgraduate students, or those working in industry or any other profession – who are teaching students from any healthcare profession.

The first chapter, 'Introducing teaching and learning', presents some of the benefits and challenges you may face as a new teacher in the healthcare professions. It provides you with a brief overview of the key principles behind teaching and learning theories and introduces some concepts that are discussed in more detail elsewhere in the book. This chapter also explains the importance of developing a personal philosophy of teaching, with guides and top tips to help you to do this.

Chapter 2, 'Developing course material', is essential reading if you have been asked to design your own lesson or course. It takes you through some basic concepts of course design and outlines the importance of considering your own teaching style and being aware of different learning styles. It also provides you with practical tips and ideas to ensure that your lesson or course meets the needs of your students.

If you are wondering how you will deliver your teaching, look no further than Chapter 3 on 'Teaching strategies and approaches to learning'. This chapter covers many ways in which you can create learning opportunities for your students. It also gives you tips on how to maximise your students' learning through a mix of evidence-based strategies that suit different learning styles. It also provides an overview of the technologies that are currently available to aid teaching and provides advice on how to introduce them to your students.

Chapter 4, 'Assessing learning', provides an easy-to-read overview of various types of assessment that you may come across as a healthcare professions teacher, and that your students will inevitably face at some point in their academic and professional careers. It explains the benefits and challenges of different assessment methods, which will enable you to select the most appropriate for your course and your students.

As a new teacher you will want to ensure that your teaching is effective. Chapter 5, 'Evaluating teaching', suggests ways to evaluate your teaching and improve your practice on the basis of this information. This is a critical part of professional development, both for the full-time educator and for a professional with part-time teaching responsibilities.

As part of this professional development, knowing how to consider your performance is an essential skill to learn. Chapter 6, 'Reflecting on teaching and learning', guides you through the process of reflection and explains how this can help you to develop ways to improve and enhance your teaching practice.

The book provides exercises to help you apply the information to your own situation, and 'top tips' to guide you in your new venture. There are also personal views from people with teaching experience – confessing the good, the bad, and the ugly!

The contributors to this book are from varying backgrounds, some of whom have had no professional teaching training but who regularly teach healthcare students and practitioners. It is written from real experience, with practical tips and useful guides to further information and resources.

Within the text various terms have been used interchangeably. 'Teacher', 'lecturer', 'assessor', 'tutor' and 'facilitator' are all used to describe the person undertaking the teaching and responsible for the learning process. Similarly, 'students', 'learners' and 'trainees' are used to describe the recipients of your teaching. You may have been asked to teach a 'course', a 'module', a 'lecture', a 'lesson' or a 'programme' and these terms have been used throughout. A glossary of terms is also included as undoubtedly you will be confronted by a barrage of confusing vocabulary when you start teaching. Words that are included in the glossary are indicated by being **bold** type in the chapter text.

There are a variety of other resources including a template lesson plan and example evaluation forms. By having suggestions for further reading, particularly on concepts that the book has mentioned in brief detail, it is hoped that you can make further links between practice and theory, and vice versa. Signposting to resources, particularly on the internet, will also provide you with further information.

This book is not intended to be a comprehensive teaching manual. It is an easy-to-read guide to help the busy new teacher to quickly and easily understand common educational concepts, to learn how to teach effectively within the given resources, and to reflect and improve upon their own teaching practice.

Sarah Carter,
July 2011

About the editor

After completing a Masters degree in Health Psychology from University College London, Dr Sarah Carter went on to work in a multidisciplinary research team at the School of Pharmacy, University of London, where she also undertook her PhD on the behavioural impact of genetic health risk information. She now manages research projects funded by organisations such as the NHS and the National Institute for Health and Clinical Excellence. While at the School of Pharmacy she has been involved in teaching, facilitating and supervising pharmacy undergraduate students, despite having no formal teaching experience. She was the Editor of the international journal *Pharmacy Education* for six years, where she encouraged authors to submit their research and managed the process of manuscript review and editing until the publication stage.

She is also currently the General Secretary of the United Kingdom Clinical Pharmacy Association.

Abbreviations

CBD	Case-Based Discussion
CoDEG	Competency Development and Evaluation Group
CPD	continuing professional development
EMQs	extended-matching questions
GLF	General Level Framework
HEI	higher education institution
ICT	information and communication technology
LMS	Learning management system
MCQ	Multiple Choice Question
mini-CEX	Mini Clinical Evaluation Exercise
Mini-PAT	Mini Peer Assessment Tool
NHS KSF	National Health Service Knowledge and Skills Framework
OER	Open Educational Resources
OSCE	Objective Structured Clinical Examination
RITA	Record of In-Training Assessment
SDL	self-directed learning
SPRAT	Sheffield Peer Review Tool
VLEs	Virtual learning environments

Contributors

Alicia Bouldin, PhD
Associate Professor for Instructional Assessment and Advancement, School of Pharmacy, University of Mississippi, Mississippi, USA.

Tina Penick Brock, EdD
Professor of Clinical Pharmacy, School of Pharmacy, University of California, San Francisco, California, USA.

Billy Futter
Emeritus Associate Professor, Rhodes University, Grahamstown, South Africa.

Sue C Jones, PhD
Clinical Pharmacy Practice Lecturer and Academic Developer, Waterloo Campus, King's College London, UK.

Barry Jubraj, PGCEA
Lead for Work-Based Learning Support, Joint Programmes Board, School of Pharmacy, University of London & Lead Pharmacist for Academic Studies, Chelsea & Westminster Hospital NHS Foundation Trust, London, UK.

Mary Monk-Tutor, PhD
Professor of Pharmacy Administration and Director of Assessment, McWhorter School of Pharmacy, Samford University, Birmingham Alabama, USA.

Timothy Rennie, PhD
Pharmacy Course Coordinator, University of Namibia, Windhoek, Namibia.

1

Introducing teaching and learning

Alicia Bouldin and Mary Monk-Tutor

The purpose of this chapter is to provide a brief overview of teaching and learning theories and concepts that are important for teachers of healthcare students to understand. The differences between teaching in didactic versus experiential settings are also discussed, as well as the benefits and challenges that new teachers face. The chapter also explains how to align beliefs about learning with a personal philosophy of teaching.

Are you a teacher?

Health science education is provided by a diverse array of multidisciplinary professionals who are not necessarily healthcare practitioners themselves. This education occurs in many settings including in the classroom, online, and at external sites where healthcare is practised. Author and education specialist Parker Palmer says that we 'lead by word and deed simply because [we] are here doing what [we] do'. Thus, each person in the healthcare environment has the opportunity to become a role model and teacher for others simply by doing his or her work.

What is the role of a teacher?

A teacher's attitude sets the tone for learning. Thus, a teacher needs to have the personal attitudes and skills to remain committed to student learning, even in challenging interpersonal situations. Because teachers need to interact with their students in many different ways, they serve as content experts, learning facilitators, motivators, role models, performance evaluators, and mentors. Let us look briefly at each of these different roles.

Content expert and learning facilitator: Teachers facilitate their students' learning by guiding them through new tasks and knowledge. Obviously, we want students to learn from our example as a content expert. We must remember, however, that our own knowledge and skills are the result of years of education, training and experience and that each student can only begin where she or he is now – we need not judge their abilities too harshly at first.

Role model and motivator: Your students will learn many important lessons from you about things such as interacting with others and being a responsible team member simply by observing your own attitudes, knowledge, and behaviour. Whether the students learn these lessons correctly or not depends on the type of role model that you set for them. As their teacher, you will also play an important role in motivating students to identify their own learning needs, set goals for personal learning, and develop skills as lifelong learners.

Performance evaluator: Teachers assess the success of students' learning in many ways, including the use of examinations, observation of student performance in a practice site, and application of complex concepts to solve real-world problems. They also play a crucial role in helping students learn how to assess themselves and their peers in an honest and constructive way.

Mentor: Teachers play a key role in the professional socialisation of healthcare students by serving as their mentors. They help students to translate their knowledge and learning into actual practice and help students to develop attitudes and values expected of the profession. This may include providing students with advice about their future careers and emotional support as well as factual knowledge.

In addition to the roles discussed above, a teacher must be able to think systematically about the learning that needs to occur, how the learning will happen, and how the learning will be assessed. To excel in these areas, a teacher simply needs to master the use of the teaching tools that will be discussed later in the book.

How does teaching differ between the didactic and the experiential settings?

In the **didactic** (or classroom) setting, you will usually be asked to cover a specified amount of content material during a specific time period to a class that includes multiple students. Class size may vary from just a few students to over 200. Most of the challenges of teaching in the didactic environment increase with class size, and include preparation of class activities that will engage students, development of handouts with learning objectives, assessment of student learning, classroom management, and in some cases, management of technology such as computers, projectors, overhead machines, sound systems, and slide screens.

The most common teaching methodology (**andragogy**) used in the didactic setting is lectures, but active learning techniques such as group projects,

Box 1.1 *What are the characteristics of a good teacher?*

It is not surprising that most good teachers have certain characteristics in common. These include 'professional' characteristics such as competence in their area of expertise, 'teacher' characteristics such as motivating students to learn, and 'human' characteristics such as an appreciation of different cultural backgrounds and a balance between their personal and professional lives.

Think back on all of your learning experiences so far. Who was your best teacher? What made this person such a good teacher? What characteristics or qualities did this person display in their teaching that you would like to emulate?

student presentations, and case-based learning may be incorporated as well (see Chapter 3). When teaching in the classroom setting, you are likely to be evaluated on your course design and organisation, classroom management, content delivery, interaction with students, approachability and other personal characteristics, ability to explain your topic, and ultimately, your ability to facilitate the learning of your students.

Compared with the didactic setting, the experiential (or practice) environment is much more dynamic because it reflects what healthcare practitioners are actually doing in the 'real world'. Those teaching in this setting must clearly identify **learning objectives** and find ways to engage students in the practice site itself, as well as assess student performance. However, the delivery of content is much more informal and less structured than in the didactic setting and is dependent on your daily responsibilities and activities in your practice setting as these will become the primary learning opportunities for your students. Common experiential learning techniques include observation, journal clubs, case presentations, and clinical activities. When teaching in the experiential setting, you are likely to be evaluated on your ability to model the knowledge and skills the student needs to learn, as well as your interaction with students and other personal characteristics, and your ability to explain your topic and facilitate your students' learning.

What are the benefits and challenges of teaching for those with little or no prior training or experience in this area?

Those with little or no formal training in teaching will certainly face some challenges. But first, let us focus on some of the benefits that you will have in your teaching. Most importantly, you are already an expert in your field and have a clear understanding of how your content area applies to healthcare practice. This content knowledge may be well ahead of what is published in your students' textbooks, since the information there is sometimes out of date by the time the book is printed. You also have the benefit of experience, which allows you to apply your knowledge in a practical way that you can explain clearly to others. Your familiarity with current standards of practice, laws and regulations, and working in multidisciplinary teams allows you to instinctively know what information is most important for students to learn about your content area and why.

Now, what about those challenges you may face? Initially, you may not have much awareness of various teaching and learning methods, theoretical models of education, or teaching tools that are available to help you. This book will help you overcome your challenges in all of those areas. However, if you are working in a healthcare practice site, your schedule may already be so overwhelming that you feel you barely have time to explain to a student what it is that you are doing, much less why you are doing it, or why you are not doing something else. Teachers in these types of settings must also overcome the challenges of the healthcare practice site itself. Some tips to help you with this appear in Appendix 1.

Education as a discipline

How do we learn?

From the moment we arrive on the planet, each of us struggles to make sense of our surroundings in the best manner we can. As we begin to make sense, we 'learn', creating knowledge. We learn that objects may be hot, that water relieves thirst, that the sky is blue, that wheels are round, and so on. Then formal education enters the picture for most of us, in an attempt to structure learning so that we are equipped with what we need to be successful participants in life, in society with others, in our callings. But while it is an important ingredient in the developmental environment, formal education does not spontaneously produce learning.

How then do people really learn? How do we process available information for future use? These are important questions to those who will be involved in the education of health professionals. And while the answers are so relevant to the success of most human undertakings, there are still no definitive explanations for what occurs in the 'black box' that is one's head when one is 'learning'.

Recent advances in brain science suggest that learning may involve some physical changes in the brain itself. Neuronal networks are the physical representation of cognitive links that are made through learning; these networks modify and grow, and they vary from person to person. When the biology of learning is considered, we may automatically look to the role that genes play in learning capacity. However, environmental factors such as nutrition, exercise, stress, emotion, and other social conditions have been examined regarding their actual influence on brain changes. Given that these non-genetic factors do indeed matter, it follows that schools, teachers, and other learning tools may have more impact than most assume.

Many theories have been postulated for understanding the cognitive aspects of learning. All were proposed in a scholarly and sincere fashion, but some are diversely opposed to others in their conceptualisation of the essential nature of learning. Among the best-known psychological theories that have been proposed to describe this phenomenon are Stimulus–Response Conditioning Theory and Cognitive Interactionist Theory. (These two leading theories are cursorily treated in this introduction; if the concepts intrigue you, please refer to the Resources section at the end of this chapter for texts that offer a more detailed examination of those and other learning theories.)

In the stimulus–response (S–R) or 'behaviourism' paradigm, it is believed that learning occurs primarily through stepwise conditioning. Stimuli (which may be arranged by a teacher) cause the subject to respond in a certain way, or at least increase the likelihood that the predicted response will occur. B.F. Skinner (1904–1990) was a prominent proponent of this theory, known generally as 'behaviourism'. Skinner and other behaviourists observed that once stimulus and response are linked in the person's brain, then positive reinforcement (e.g. reward) encourages the repetition of the response, as does negative reinforcement (e.g. removal of a negative stimulus). Behaviourists consider this change in behaviour to represent 'learning'. More repetitions are theorised to lead to greater retention of the learning. 'Learning' a piano piece for recital may be accomplished best by practice, or repetition. An example from the classroom would include 'drills' or exercises including flash cards for learning multiplication tables or chemical structures. This may explain how we learn some of the most basic elements of our knowledge. Most of us can attest to the contribution of exercises and practised responses to stimuli in our own learning journey. However, the other major field of learning theory suggests that behaviourism does not tell the whole story.

Reflection or pursuit of insight is another way of conceptualising 'learning'. Proponents of the cognitive interactional theory posit that learning occurs as insight is acquired or as thoughts are modified through experience. Many may be familiar with the quotation 'experience is the best teacher'. Whether or not one agrees that it is the 'best' teacher, one must certainly agree that experience does provide opportunity for learning. According to this paradigm, it is the interaction between the individual and his or her environment that generates the cognitive work that makes learning occur; we interact with and reflect on things until they 'make sense'. (Refer to Chapter 6 regarding reflection as an integral part of learning in the health professions.) This is deemed by some to be a more progressive approach to understanding what occurs as we learn or process information.

This 'learn by doing' maxim has been applied in health education, and may be reflected in teaching methods such as **problem-based learning** (which is discussed more in Chapter 3) and **experiential learning**, the latter of which is a component of virtually all health professions education, regardless of discipline. It is one thing to 'know about' the use of a sphyg-momanometer to measure blood pressure; but it is quite another thing to 'know how' to do it accurately and well. (In fact, some may find it difficult to learn without 'doing'; more discussion on learning styles may be found in Chapter 2.)

The concept of learning by doing has been expanded in recent years to include **service learning**, in which experiential learning occurs in a context that provides a simultaneous service to others. For example, pharmacy students may develop a deeper understanding of the effect of socioeconomic factors on patient regimen adherence by volunteering at a free clinic and reflecting on the experience. Another benefit of learning certain knowledge or skills in a service-oriented context is the possibility that one may also learn desirable attitudes, such as empathy and compassion.

Which of these theories best describes your own understanding of what it means to learn? Your understanding of how learning occurs will certainly influence your approach to teaching. As a teacher, one of your primary roles will be to foster learning, to motivate students to process and retain information. Your own understanding of information processing will be a primary factor in how you design the learning environment for those you teach.

How do we teach?

With a more progressive approach towards understanding learning, thoughts on teaching have begun to change also (see Fig. 1.1). The 'sage on the stage' image is giving way to the picture of a facilitative 'guide on the side', as our approach towards teaching shifts from teacher-centred, where students were dependent vessels waiting to be filled, to **learner-centred**, where the student is an independent learner, constructing knowledge from a variety of sources (one of which is certainly the teacher).

Just as there are many learning theories that try to explain the 'black box' of learning, there are a variety of teaching approaches that have been tried. Each has some value, and perhaps some more than others in given contexts. If general categories of teaching methods may be considered to reside on a continuum, from teacher-centred to learner-centred, the result might resemble Fig. 1.2.

An overview of these general categories as they relate to the continuum is described here; later chapters address the specifics of course design (Chapter 2) and the use of teaching strategies (Chapter 3).

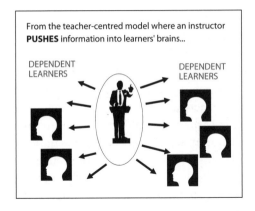

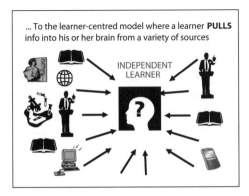

Figure 1.1. Teacher-centred versus learner-centred learning.

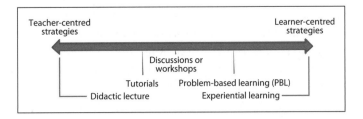

Figure 1.2. Teaching methods on a teaching approach continuum.

The basic didactic lecture is perhaps in principle the most teacher-centred method in use at present. This is not to say that there is no place for the didactic approach, where a lecturer 'professes' information to a large group of students. Even that educational setting may provide opportunities for active learning and learner application of newly constructed knowledge if the class environment is organised by the teacher to encourage such behaviours. Obviously, basic knowledge of the informational sort may be acquired through the efficient and often effective lecture mode. However, additional andragogies are being employed in today's healthcare education to enable development of necessary skills and attitudes (such as lifelong learning) in addition to knowledge.

Discussion as a teaching method can be a very effective blend of teacher-centred and learner-centred foci. The instructor may still relate information and guide the path that further discussion follows. But as students participate openly in questions, answers, and presentation of their own ideas related to the learning topics, they become more active constructors of their own knowledge and skills. Involving other learners in the information being shared also enhances collaborative learning opportunities among peers. Professionals often engage in peer discussions in real environments, to build or correct their understandings. In this way, building discussion skills early in one's educational programme may serve to facilitate lifelong learning.

In healthcare education, the use of cases has become a standard curricular element. **Case-based** teaching provides learners with the opportunity to engage with the material and apply what they know or have learned. Cases supplement the more traditional lectures, and are flexible enough to be employed within a classroom setting (especially 'mini-cases') or outside, for self-directed learning. Cases often make basic information seem more relevant, and thus can increase the motivation to learn content explored through this method, which is discussed in more detail in Chapter 3.

Problem-based learning (PBL) is a form of active learning in which learners are presented with complex scenarios in which they must identify and correctly solve the problems that exist. This usually involves group-based work, so that the learning occurs collaboratively. The approach is very student-centred, but is facilitated by a tutor or instructor. When PBL activities are structured well, enabling learner guidance and support, students generally respond enthusiastically to the opportunity to construct new and adaptive knowledge, while exercising their thinking skills and working together to reach a solution. In theory, application of skills and knowledge in this fashion is likely to result in learning that lasts. Learners are actively engaged with the problem, and with each other, so teachers employing this technique need to be aware of the potential effects of group dynamics on the learning environment.

Experiential learning is perhaps the most learner-centred approach in which the teacher is still present. It is highly appealing to those who learn best by doing. It has obvious advantages in health professions education, where in many ways it mimics the oldest form of professional education—the apprenticeship. Today's experiential learning provides students the opportunity to be mentored (individually or in very small groups) through real (or simulated) situations in which their knowledge and skills are directly applied. Demonstrating one's learning is highly rewarding both to learner and teacher alike, building confidence in skills and knowledge.

Service learning may be thought of as 'off' the continuum. It is highly learner-centred, but also 'others'-centred. In this method students learn by participating in and reflecting on activities that meet an identified need in the community. Applying learning in a real-world environment while community-based others are helped through the learning experience may facilitate the achievement of several broad outcomes: learning and applying curricular content, developing or fostering a service orientation (attitude), and giving back to the community in a meaningful way. Both learners and teachers generally derive some internal reward from participation in this fashion.

The foundation of critical thinking

Whatever the method employed, one reason for the impetus behind education that is more learner-centred is the essential need for the ability of critical thinking. The concept of critical thinking is a relatively complex one, and may be distilled to mean a reasoned consideration of evidence, or reflectively making sound judgements. This is directly applicable to health professions education. Cognitive skills are required to think critically or analytically, of course. But critical thinking also entails a philosophy, a willingness to reflect and apply advanced thinking to problems that arise.

As teachers, to foster critical thinking we must provide an environment in which students can safely explore their intellectual curiosity about learning topics. We should allow the questions 'why?' and 'how?' and then engage learners in pursuit of the answers by thinking – real thinking – that involves judgement and pondering. They may need some guidance at first, as the higher-order thinking skills of analysis and synthesis are all too easy to avoid in both learning and teaching. It requires effort for the learner to think critically, and in truth it requires effort to structure teaching so that critical thinking on the part of the learner is necessary. But the benefits are certainly worth the hard work. As one gains practice in resolving inquiries that require critical thinking, one's confidence in one's reasoning ability increases. And both skill and confidence in reasoning and judgement are essential components of the health professional's toolkit.

Learner-centred technologies

Learner-centred methods, simulations, critical thinking, self-directed learning: many of the concepts that are currently being promoted in health professions education can be facilitated through innovative use of technology. For today's learners, technology also has the potential to increase internal motivation to learn, if only because they enjoy the interactive nature of the

Box 1.2 Some technology tools for teaching

- PowerPoint
- Animations
- Simulations
- Personal response systems ('clickers')
- PDAs, smartphones
- Games
- Flashcards
- Podcasts (audio and video)
- Weblogs, wikis
- Web conferencing
- Remote video, streaming video
- Social networking
- Interactive white board
- Independent study, online courses

technology-enhanced task. That motivation for some is enhanced because the technology helps to address diverse learning styles with appeal to multiple learning preferences simultaneously: visual, auditory, kinaesthetic, and verbal. (See Chapter 2 for more on learning styles.)

Technology has been applied in a variety of ways to educational ends. (See Chapter 3 for a discussion on the concept of elearning, or applying technology to distance learning.) Commonly technology is used within the classroom to supplement or enhance content delivery; videos or personal response devices ('clickers') are examples of this use. Similar supplements and enhancements may be employed outside of class, providing basic supporting information as well as links or exercises for further exploration of material. And the broadest use of technology in teaching is through online classes, both synchronous and asynchronous. Chapter 3 discusses teaching methods in which technology may be useful.

If technology tools (see Box 1.2) are used to complement the teaching method, they have the ability to make learning more meaningful by compounding the individual or collaborative experience.

However, teachers should be cautioned not to use technology 'for the sake of it'. Excessive or unnecessary use of technology provides no significant benefit to teacher or learner. In addition, not all learners have access to all forms of technology. So, when making instructional technology choices, match the tools to your needs and those of your learners. Examine the learning or instructional goals you have set: What do you expect to learn, or expect your students to learn? What skills and knowledge should be acquired? Also examine the setting in which the learning is to take place: Will the learner be at home? In the office? In a clinical setting? In a lecture hall? The answers to these questions should drive the use of the technology. The medium is not the message.

Examining our learning and our teaching

When we engage in conversation with friends, or in consultation with patients, the only way to know whether our message has been accurately perceived is through feedback from the patient or the conversational partner. That feedback may be verbal or non-verbal, may be formal or informal, may be interjected in the middle of our message or at the end. But unless we have some indication from the other, we have no evidence that our message has been received in the way we intended.

Likewise, in education, one must have some feedback to ensure that the desired learning has taken place. As we rarely find ourselves in informal conversation with each individual student about every learning topic, this feedback occurs most commonly through formal assessments of learning.

Chapter 4 of this book relates the particulars of a variety of assessment techniques. We are all familiar with the use of examinations as formal and often summative assessments of learning. But in addition to **summative assessments**, it may be argued that **formative assessments** (which inform the learner of their current progress) are key in order for assessment to be as meaningful as possible in the learner-centred educational model. In addition, self-assessment on the part of the learner is an important component, and one that is a critical skill for lifelong learning. Learners need to be able to evaluate their own progress, observe gaps in knowledge or skills, and lay out a plan for continued growth.

Learning portfolios are an excellent tool to support both learning and teaching. Such portfolios are a collection of evidence of learning, arranged in an organised fashion to support the observation of the learner's growth over time. This concept combines formative assessment with self-assessment and reflection, yielding a forum for the individual learner to explore their own learning and observe their progress. It is valuable for the teacher to review this as well, as the insight provided by this direct observation of artefacts may enable formative feedback and guidance. Portfolios are of particular value in experiential learning, where the students' documentation of various learning outcomes serves as a virtual 'journal' of their performance, and even of learning that is otherwise not directly observable (attitude change, for example). Both the student and teacher/evaluator benefit from the availability of this reflective examination of the learning that occurred.

Examining our teaching is just as important as the examination of learning. While some aspects of our teaching may be evaluated through the performance of our students, there are other meaningful mechanisms through which feedback may be gathered in relation to our performance as teachers. Some of those means are external (feedback provided by others who reflect on our teaching), and some internal (our own reflections on our teaching). All are useful if done with an eye towards enabling improvement. Chapter 5 expands upon the use of opinions from others to improve teaching, and Chapter 6 provides guidance for self-reflection.

How can teaching and learning theories be used to improve your teaching?

What does the above information from the experiences of educational philosophers and psychological and physiological forums mean to the rank-and-file teacher/mentor/facilitator? Taken collectively, it can help us to develop our own understanding of what it means to learn, and thereby influence our philosophies of how we will then teach others. If we have a philosophy—a foundational guide for our decisions in teaching—and are not just flying blind, then we can observe progress and understand what is not working and what to change. Establishing a 'teaching philosophy' is rather like having an exercise or diet plan based on a philosophy of living. You might adjust it on the basis of outcome, but it is a foundational start. Keep in mind that your personal teaching philosophy will likely change over time as you mature and become a more experienced teacher.

What is a personal philosophy of teaching?

A **philosophy of teaching** is a formal written document that addresses the questions 'Why do I teach?' and 'How do I believe people learn?' As such, it serves as a reflection on your personal implicit and explicit assumptions about teaching and learning. Its purpose is to identify and guide your teaching goals and teaching methods, and also to communicate this information to others. For example, many schools require the submission of a personal teaching philosophy when applying for a job in academia.

How, then, does one describe one's teaching philosophy to others? It is one thing to 'say' you have a general philosophy about how you will teach, but it is another to actually have one formally described. The latter is very valuable as it brings into focus the reflective self-assessment needed to seriously consider one's role in the learning of others, whether those others are students, peers, or even family. While there is no single 'correct' format or content for a teaching philosophy, it is helpful to review the philosophies of other teachers prior to preparing your own. Look in the Resources section at the end of this chapter for examples of teaching philosophies.

How do I prepare a philosophy of teaching?

Preparing a teaching philosophy requires personal introspection and reflection, and thus is a process that will take differing amounts of time for different people. You may need to prepare multiple drafts to capture your thoughts about what is most important to you about teaching and learning. Remember that *your* philosophy is just that – it is yours. As such, it cannot be incorrect. It should clearly reflect who you are as a teacher right now, not what you think someone else wants to hear or what you think you should believe about teaching and learning.

A teaching philosophy is typically short (one or two typed pages maximum) and unique to you (and thus written in the first person voice). Initially, your philosophy may be somewhat idealistic, but it will likely become more practical with each revision and with the maturation of your teaching skills. For a walk-through on how to articulate your own philosophy of teaching, see Appendix 2.

How do you evaluate your personal philosophy of teaching?

Writing down your teaching philosophy helps to clarify your thinking about teaching and learning and allows you to become more aware of why you teach the way that you do. More specifically, the process encourages you to review your teaching priorities (and reorganise them, if necessary), rethink your teaching strategies and learning activities and their effectiveness, and continue to plan for your future growth as a teacher. Over time, this type of reflection may help you to identify philosophical shifts in your teaching or needs for revisions in your teaching goals or pedagogies.

As with other teaching activities, periodic self-reflection and evaluation of your philosophy is a useful exercise. It is not a static document, so do not hesitate to make changes to it over time. You will probably want to review it at least every two to three years and make any necessary updates based on your current beliefs about teaching and learning at the time. As you review the document, ask yourself 'How well does my written teaching philosophy capture and communicate my current feelings about teaching and learning?' It may also be helpful to have others review your philosophy (see Box 1.3).

Conclusion

Now that you have some foundational information, you can start the journey to becoming a better teacher. The following chapters in this book will guide you through the steps of designing your course or other learning experience, developing learning aims and outcomes for your content material, and understanding and adapting to different learning styles of your students

Box 1.3 *Evaluating your teaching philosophy*

Based on a review of the teaching philosophy, answer the following questions.

1 What does the writer most value about teaching and learning? How do you know?
2 Does the writer identify a clear teaching style? What is it?
3 Does the writer seem confident and comfortable with his/her ideas about teaching and learning? What words in the document support your answer?
4 Does reading the philosophy help you to understand how and why the writer teaches as he/she does? How so?
5 What part of this writer's philosophy seems most relevant to his/her discipline or expertise?
6 What is most memorable to you about the writer's philosophy? Why?
7 What is most unclear to you about the writer's philosophy? How could it be improved?
8 What do you like most about the writer's philosophy? Why?

(Chapter 2). Chapter 3 takes you through different methods of teaching and provides excellent tips on how to use these methods to engage your learners. While the evaluation of your teaching may seem intimidating, it is an important element in the journey, as it facilitates improvement and provides direction for continued forward motion. So stand ready to assess the product of your teaching (Chapter 4), intentionally use that evaluation data to improve your teaching (Chapter 5), and engage in self-reflection on your teaching (Chapter 6).

Choosing to embrace your role as teacher and seeking professional development through resources such as this book are two important steps along the path. But be reminded that there are many others who are walking this path at the same time. The role of teacher is as old as the most basic of human relationships, and the experience of other teachers will hold valuable lessons for you. So try not to take on this journey in isolation. Be encouraged to interact with peers and mentors, exploring the ways in which your efforts may make the most difference to those who learn from you, either directly or indirectly. For knowing that you have made a difference is the greatest reward.

References and further reading

Bigge ML, Shermis SS (1999). *Learning Theories for Teachers*, 6th edn. New York: Longman.

Center for Effective Teaching and Learning at the University of Texas at El Paso (CETaL). *Articulating Your Philosophy of Teaching*. http://sunconference.utep.edu/CETaL/resources/portfolios/writetps.htm#comments (accessed 25 March 2010).

Center for Instructional Development and Research. *Writing Tips to Help You Get Started on a Teaching Portfolio: Drafting a Teaching Statement*. http://depts.washington.edu/cidrweb/resources/writingtips.html (accessed 26 March 2010).

Chickering A, Gamson Z (1987). Seven principles of good practice in undergraduate education. *AAHE Bulletin* **39**: 3–7.

Chism NV (1997–1998). Developing a philosophy of teaching statement. *Essays on Teaching Excellence: Toward the Best in the Academy 9.3*.

Fascione PA (2010). *Critical Thinking: What It Is and Why It Counts (2010 Update)*. Millbrae, CA: California Academic Press. www.insightassessment.com/pdf_files/what&why2009.pdf (accessed 22 March 2010).

Goodyear GE, Alichin D (1998). Statements of teaching philosophy. In: Kaplan M, ed. *To Improve the Academy, 17*. Stillwater, OK: New Forums Press and the Professional and Organizational Development Network in Higher Education, 103–122.

Haugen L (1988). *Writing a Teaching Philosophy Statement*. Ames, IA: Center for Teaching Excellence, Iowa State University. www.celt.iastate.edu/teaching/philosophy.html (accessed 26 March 2010).

Jensen EP (2008). A Fresh Look at Brain-Based Education. *Phi Delta Kappan* **89**(6): 408–417.

King A (1993). From Sage on the Stage to Guide on the Side. *College Teaching* **41**(1): 30–35.

Monk-Tutor MR *et al.* (2007). Development of a service-learning component in a required course in fiscal management. *Journal of Pharmacy Teaching* **14**(2): 23–54.

Murray JP (1995). *Successful Faculty Development and Evaluation. The Complete Teaching Portfolio* (ASHE-ERIC Higher Education Report No 8). Washington, DC: The George Washington University, Graduate School of Education and Human Development.

National Board for Professional Teaching Standards. *What Teachers Should Know and Be Able to Do*. Arlington, VA: NBPTS. www.nbpts.org/UserFiles/File/what_teachers.pdf (accessed 23 March 2010).

Palmer P (2000). *Let Your Life Speak: Listening for the Voice of Vocation*. New York: Wiley.

Popovich NG *et al.* (2010). Eliminating bottlenecks to learning among pharmacy students. *American Journal of Pharmaceutical Education* **74**(1). www.aacp.org (accessed 07 March 2010).

Rhem J (1998). Problem-based Learning: An Introduction. *The National Teaching & Learning FORUM* **8**(1). www.ntlf.com/html/pi/9812/pbl_1.htm (accessed 22 March 2010).

Seldin P (1997). *The Teaching Portfolio: A Practical Guide to Improved Performance and Promotion/Tenure Decisions*, 2nd edn. Bolton, MA: Anker Publishing.

Sutkin G *et al.* (2008). What makes a good clinical teacher in medicine? A review of the literature. *Academic Medicine* **83**(5): 452–466.

Western University of Health Sciences and American Association of Colleges of Pharmacy (2010). *Education Scholar Module 1: Developing a Personal Working Philosophy to Guide Teaching/Learning in the Health Professions Education*. Available online at www.educationscholar.org (accessed 22 March 2010).

Western University of Health Sciences and American Association of Colleges of Pharmacy (2010). *Education Scholar Module 2: Facilitating Learning in a Traditional Classroom Setting*. Available online at www.educationscholar.org (accessed 22 March 2010).

Western University of Health Sciences and American Association of Colleges of Pharmacy (2010). *Education Scholar Module 3: Improving Outcomes through the Use of Active Learning Strategies*. Available online at www.educationscholar.org (accessed 22 March 2010).

Western University of Health Sciences and American Association of Colleges of Pharmacy (2010). *Education Scholar Module 4C: Learning in the Experiential Setting*. Available online at www.educationscholar.org (accessed 22 March 2010).

Zubizaretta J (2004). *The Learning Portfolio: Reflective Practice for Improving Student Learning*. Boston, MA: Anker Publishing.

Zull JE (2002). *The Art of Changing the Brain: Enriching the Practice of Teaching by Exploring the Biology of Learning*. Sterling, VA: Stylus Publishing.

Resources

Bransford JD *et al.* eds. (2000). *How People Learn: Brain, Mind, Experience and School*. Washington, DC: National Academy Press.

Campus Compact. *Service-learning: Using structured reflection to enhance learning from service*. Available online at: www.compact.org/disciplines/reflection (accessed 11 March 2011).

Campus Technology. http://campustechnology.com/Home.aspx (accessed 11 March 2011).

Curry L, Wergin JF (1993). *Educating Professionals: Responding to New Expectations and Accountability*. San Francisco, CA: Jossey-Bass Publishers.

Davis BG (1993). *Tools for Teaching*. San Francisco: Jossey-Bass.

Kearsley G (2011). *The Theory Into Practice Database: Explorations in Learning and Instruction*. http://tip.psychology.org/ (accessed 11 March 2011).

Llewellyn DC (2004). *Glossary of Learning Terms*. http://www.cetl.gatech.edu/resources/learningterms.pdf (accessed 11 March 2011).

Lourdes CM, Ginsburg DB (2005). *Preceptor's Handbook for Pharmacists*. Bethesda, MD: ASHP.

McKeachie WJ, Svinicki M, eds. (2006). *McKeachie's Teaching Tips: Strategies, Research, and Theory for College and University Teachers*, 12th edn. Boston, MA: Houghton Mifflin.

Schumann W *et al.* (2004). Integrating service and reflection in the professional development of pharmacy students. *American Journal of Pharmaceutical Education* 68(2). www.ajpe.org/view.asp?art=aj680245&pdf=yes (accessed 11 March 2011).

The Carnegie Foundation for the Advancement of Teaching: The Knowledge Media Laboratory (KML). http://www.carnegiefoundation.org/previous-work/knowledge-media-lab (accessed 11 March 2011).

University of Minnesota CEHD (2010). *Resources for Teachers: Portfolios*. College of Education and Human Development. Available online at www.cehd.umn.edu/career/teacher/default.html (accessed 24 March 2010).

2

Developing course material

Sue C Jones and Billy Futter

If you have been asked to teach healthcare students it is most likely that the curriculum, course or programme is already established. However, sometimes you may be asked to design your own course or module, or add elements to an existing course. This chapter takes you through some basic concepts of planning and design to ensure that your course meets the needs of your learners.

What is involved in course design?

When planning and designing a lesson or course, key questions you will need to address are:

- *Aims:* Why am I teaching this course?
- *Objectives:* What should the students know or be able to do after the course? Will they achieve increased insight, understanding and awareness; informed attitudes and opinions; improved professional or technical ability, or interpersonal skills?
- *Audience:* What do I know about my audience? What is their existing ability, what have they learnt prior to this, and what are their expectations? What is their learning style? How motivated are they to learn?
- *Materials:* What supplies, media and other equipment do I need in order to teach the course? What materials do the students need?
- *Time:* How much time do I have? How much time do the students have (for example, hours per week) for my course and other courses?
- *Teaching methods:* Which teaching method(s) will most likely achieve the desired outcomes within the resource and audience constraints? (See Chapter 3.)
- *Assessment:* How will I know whether the learning outcomes have been achieved? For example, what assessment criteria and methods will I use? (See Chapter 5.)
- *Evaluation:* What do I need to do differently to improve the teaching session next time? (See Chapter 4.)

Learning aims, objectives and outcomes

Most higher education institutions (HEIs) plan and design their courses around learning aims, objectives and outcomes. You will be required by your institution to specify these when designing your course. They are helpful in focusing and organising your thoughts in order to design high-quality material. They will also ensure that any added content is actually required. By retaining focus at this level, your students will achieve a clear awareness of what is expected.

Learning aims

This is a good starting point when writing a new course. A **learning aim** is fairly general and strategic – usually a couple of sentences describing what you, as the teacher, intend to cover in the course. For example, the learning aim for a drug discovery module may be *to develop an appreciation and classification of the chemical and biological technologies used in the drug discovery process.*

Learning objectives

You may also come across the term **learning objective**. Learning objectives are more focused, specific statements of learning intention. For each learning aim, therefore, there will be several learning objectives. Continuing with the example of a drug discovery module, one example would be *to compare the role of different genera of plants in the drug discovery process.*

It is worth noting that learning objectives can be written from both the teaching point of view and the learning point of view. This lack of consistency in definitions has led to some institutions abandoning the use of learning objectives in their course descriptions and using the term 'learning outcomes' instead.

Learning outcomes

Learning outcomes are clear statements of what the learner is expected to achieve when they have completed the course, and how they are expected to have demonstrated their achievements. For example, *identify and critique valid scientific literature in the area of drug discovery; write a scientifically based report on drug discovery aspects using available academic and scientific literature.*

How to write learning aims and outcomes

Learning involves different levels of complexity. As learners progress they move on to a more complex level of learning. Fig. 2.1 shows that the simplest level is the remembering of facts, moving through to the ability to apply those facts, analyse and ultimately create ideas.

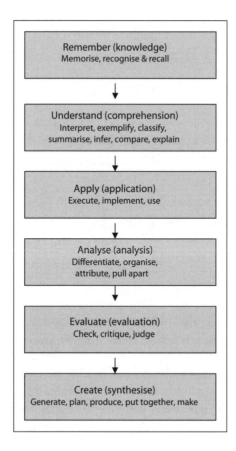

Figure 2.1. Bloom's taxonomy of learning. (Adapted from Bloom 1956; Krathwohl 2002.)

Consider these levels of learning, and use the verbs to help you write your learning aims and outcomes.

Note that the diagram considers only the knowledge, or cognitive, domain. Although this is the one that most people focus on when writing learning outcomes, you may also need to consider affective and psycho motor domains. Affective domains would include values and attitudes. These may be useful, for example, in an ethics course. The psychomotor domain would cover physical learning outcomes. You may want to consider this area if you are teaching physical clinical skills such as administering vaccinations.

Are your learning outcomes SMART?

Another way to think about your learning outcomes is by using the SMART acronym. Are they **S**pecific? Are they **M**easurable and **A**chievable? Are they **R**ealistic? Can they be delivered within yours and your students' Timeframe?

A non-SMART learning outcome might be:

Write a report on drug discovery.

By adding in a few key words it can become SMART:

By the end of this course you will be able to write a 3000-word scientifically based report on drug discovery aspects using available academic and scientific literature.

Your audience

Knowing your audience – their existing knowledge, their expectations and preferred styles of learning – will help guide you in terms of the level at which you should aim the course.

Learning styles

There are many sites on the internet where you and your students can take a test to find out about **learning styles** (see Resources at the end of the chapter).

By reading about each style you will be able to appreciate the potential differences among your students and how they respond to different teaching strategies. Doing this will allow you to ensure that your course materials will engage all types of learner, whatever their learning style.

Most people have a dominant learning style. Think of your personal preference. For example, do you learn best when presented with:

- Visual information – diagrams, graphs, mind maps, well-illustrated PowerPoint presentations?
- Aural information – clearly explained meanings, discussions and tutorials (rather than having to read a book)?
- Reading or writing – notes, reference books, written summaries on PowerPoint?
- Experiences – working with reality, case studies, and opportunities to do things?

Preferred learning styles will vary between your students. From a practical point of view, accept that it is not possible to cater for all learning styles. However, making sure you know your own preferred learning style may help you when teaching (see Personal view 2.1).

Make sure that you do not rely on one particular style, be it visual (pictures and handouts), verbal (lectures or discussion groups) or active learning tasks. A mix of different approaches will ensure you appeal to your whole audience, and will also enrich the learning experience for everyone.

Personal view 2.1

When I started teaching I was asked to deliver ten lectures on the law relating to medical practice. I had studied this as an undergraduate and really struggled with it. I hated reading the books so I was dreading the task of trying to teach such a dull subject to the students.

I spoke to the person who had done this previously and they gave me their handouts. It reminded me of my days at university. Reams and reams of written facts under headings with each word merging into another; I started to get anxious.

Once I had gathered my thoughts I sat down and drew some mind maps to help me to remember links between legislation and medical concepts. As I saw the links I could visualise how to teach it. I realised that I am someone who likes pictures to illustrate the facts, that my preferred learning style is visual. By using this as a strength I could see my way through the problem.

Mei-li, teacher practitioner

Teaching styles

You may have come across the terms **deep learning approach** and **surface learning approach**. Educators now know that students will remember information better if they engage with the material in a deeper way and take the time to fully immerse themselves in their learning. Conversely, a surface approach to learning (such as rote learning) is seen as superficial, and does not allow for learning how to use or integrate the concepts taught.

In order for students to fully understand your course, you can adopt approaches that encourage a deeper understanding. There are four main ways to do this (Biggs 1989):

1 *Student motivation*
   Students need to be motivated and engaged in their learning for it to be effective. Case studies and problem-based learning help to provide context and relevance for students. You should also consider the physical environment and teaching space. Make sure that the room you are teaching in is suitable – that is, at a comfortable temperature, well lit and arranged so that it is easy for everyone to see presentations.

2 *Learner activities*
   Getting students to actively participate in the course will encourage deeper learning. Introduce role-plays or discussion groups – learning

with peers can embed theory into practice. Students are more likely to remember information this way, rather than being passive recipients of the course.

3 *Interactions with others*

Working on specific tasks in collaboration with team mates and/or the teacher will encourage deeper learning.

4 *Integrating knowledge*

By contextualising the information, students can see where it 'fits' within their existing knowledge, and will understand better its relevance and application. Illustrating theory with case studies and examples that are relevant to the students is a very valuable tool for learning.

Teaching and learning resources

Resources are needed to equip your teaching environment. We may sometimes take for granted the availability of audiovisual equipment, for example for a presentation projected from a computer or an overhead projector (OHP). However, resource limitations may destroy all your good intentions to teach in a particular manner, so it is vital to confirm what will be available in the day-to-day situation of teaching in advance. You may need to modify how you manage your teaching in light of what is available for use.

To be prepared you may wish to keep handy a box with general items that you may need in the classroom: acetates, OHP pens, self-adhesive notes, paper. In addition, it is worth thinking about emergency situations when equipment might not be available. What is your contingency plan?

Money may be scarce. For example, a budget may be needed for consumables or for paying tutorial assistants. Remember that students also have expenses such as printing costs, buying books and internet access.

You may be expected to work within significant time constraints (see Box 2.1). You will also need to consider the students' time constraints. They will be studying independently, preparing for writing assignments, readings and assessments, for your course and other courses.

Avoid the temptation to cater for your top or bottom students. The former are quick to grasp concepts, so if the course is delivered at their level even the average student would struggle to keep up. Focusing on your less-capable students may slow down the rest of the group, who may feel unchallenged.

Also, try to prevent an unbalanced programme in which one course places an unfair time commitment on the students, to the detriment of other courses. This is where carefully written and executed learning aims and objectives can help.

Box 2.1 Time-consuming tasks to consider

- Developing teaching materials (reading material, references, case studies, MS Powerpoint presentations, self-assessment opportunities)
- Delivering the learning material and engaging with the students (lectures, online discussions, emails, tutorials)
- Providing feedback for assessment exercises (case studies, essays, debates, portfolios, reflective writing)
- Administrative issues associated with teaching and learning (e.g. booking rooms, timetabling, booking data projectors, recording performance and reporting for quality assurance purposes)
- Evaluation, review, reflection and improvement (e.g. review of curriculum in response to changing needs, technology)
- Keeping up with your discipline specialisation and the topics for which you have teaching responsibility (e.g. reading research papers, reviewing new textbooks and web sites, conducting and supervising research, submitting research papers for publication, conference presentations)

Who else needs to be involved with course design?

When designing a course there are several other groups of people or individuals whom you may wish to involve. Your line manager or head of department will have a strategic vision of how they see the course developing and how it integrates with other courses. Discuss your plans with them to ensure that your course fits within the wider programme of learning. You may also have to consider national or international guidelines. Here the need to meet accreditation standards or manage the process of having assigned academic 'credits' or 'points' to learning may need to be considered (see Box 2.2).

You could also consult an experienced teacher who has designed course material before. They will inevitably have some useful advice for you.

The students' or learners' voice is vital: they can give you their perspective, which is often neglected.

Are there any other people who may have useful information for you? For example, if you are designing a course about communicating with patients, then it would be good to talk to someone from this group.

What are all these people going to do?

Now that you have thought about the people who can influence and be influenced by your new course, you might find it useful to think about their

Box 2.2 *Official guidelines to consider*

When designing a course you may need to refer to some official documentation to ensure that the course is fit for purpose. For example, many degree courses in the UK have Quality Assurance Agency (www.qaa.ac.uk) benchmark statements, and the ACPE in the United States ensures quality for pharmacy education (www. acpe-accredit.org).

While you may not be developing a whole degree (if you are then we would suggest a different book!) you may find these resources useful. Also, if your subject is very precise then you will need to ensure that you have the most accurate and up-to-date advice, guidelines or information to populate the course content.

Bear in mind that your institution may have a standard process that you will be required to follow. Here you will need to seek specialist regulations advice from your particular institution.

roles and responsibilities. Make sure you know what your responsibility is for the course. If you have a team of people to help, such as administrators, teaching assistants or practitioners, are they clear about their roles and responsibilities? And do not forget the students – ensure that they know exactly what is expected of them during the course.

How do you want to teach your course?

Having decided on clear aims and objectives, and considered your audience, you need to think about the best way to deliver the course. Chapter 3 provides information and advice on teaching methods and strategies.

Assessment of the learning outcomes

You will also need to consider how to ensure that the learners have met the learning outcomes for the course you have designed. Read Chapter 4 for information on how to include appropriate methods of assessment in your course.

Planning your 'To Do' list

Planning is key in teaching. When developing new teaching material you would be wise to allow around 7 hours for every formal hour of teaching. If you need information from others, give them plenty of time to prepare it for you. Deadlines are vital to ensure that the course is prepared and ready in time. It can be useful to work backwards from the last deadline and map the tasks against the time available.

Think about writing a lesson plan. This will help you structure what you want to achieve in the course, what you want the students to learn, and the resources required. Keep it short, simple and easy to use, and leave space to write notes on your evaluation of the teaching session afterwards. See Appendix 3 for a template lesson plan, and a weblink under Resources at the end of this chapter.

When thinking about your to-do list, you can use project planning tools to help. You could create yourself a simple table such as the one below:

Task	Who is responsible?	Deadline

Alternatively, you could use other tools such as a Fishbone diagram or a Gantt chart (see Resources at the end of the chapter for weblinks to these tools).

Finally, do not forget the administrative side of running a course. Ensure that your course is timetabled correctly, that rooms are booked for teaching, and that handouts are photocopied or emailed.

Plagiarism

There is much debate around detecting and punishing plagiarism. However, the notion of plagiarism is often embedded in the culture of the institution within which students are being taught. It could be argued that all students when engaging in learning are 'culturally' naive to the rules and regulations around plagiarism. Therefore, initially, it is the responsibility of both teachers and learners to be aware of plagiarism and to know how to avoid it. Additionally, as educators it is our role and duty to ensure that our students have a learning environment or course design that minimises opportunities for plagiarism; for example, by changing assessments every year or by designing an assessment that is sufficiently robust to minimise plagiarism. Chapter 4 will assist you in the design of robust assessment methods.

Summary

Designing a course is challenging, but ultimately rewarding. This chapter has guided you through the essential components of course design and warned you of potential difficulties. You will find the subsequent chapters in this book on teaching and learning strategies, assessment, evaluation and reflection, essential to complement what you have learned here.

A well-designed course will be a credit to you, with both you and your students benefiting from your hard work.

Top tips

- Once you start teaching, try to talk to a variety of people who design courses to get a range of practical tips on what to do.
- Planning is vital when designing courses.
- If you find you are thrown in at the deep end, be organised and work through your 'to do' list as soon as you can.
- Do not underestimate the time it will take to develop course materials. If you are working as a team it can take longer unless you have a consensus of ideas and opinions.

References and further reading

Biggs JB (1989). Approaches to the enhancement of tertiary teaching. *Higher Education Research and Development* 8(1): 7–25.

Bloom BS, ed. (1956). *Taxonomy of Educational Objectives, The Classification of Educational Goals – Handbook I: Cognitive Domain*. New York: McKay.

Krathwohl DR (2002). A revision of Bloom's taxonomy: An overview. *Theory into Practice* 41(4): 212–218.

Carroll J (2002). *A Handbook for Deterring Plagiarism in Higher Education*. Oxford: Oxford Centre for Staff and Learning Development.

Leask B (2006). Plagiarism, cultural diversity and metaphor – implications for academic staff development. *Assessment & Evaluation in Higher Education* 31(2): 183–199.

For more information on overall course design

Toohey S (1999). *Designing Courses for Higher Education*. Buckingham: Open University Press.

All HEIs throughout the European Higher Education Area must conform to the requisite of the Bologna Agreement that all modules and programmes should be (re)written in terms of learning outcomes. This document provides extensive advice on how to do this

Kennedy D *et al.* (2003). *Writing and Using Learning Outcomes: a Practical Guide* [online]. www.bologna.msmt.cz/files/learning-outcomes.pdf (accessed 25 February 2011).

How to construct and use mind maps

www.buzanworld.com/Mind_Maps.htm
http://freemind.sourceforge.net/wiki/index.php/Main_Page

For more information on learning styles

VARK Learning styles: www.vark-learn.com
www.ldpride.net/learningstyles.MI.htm
www.engr.ncsu.edu/learningstyles/ilsweb.html

For help writing a lesson plan

www.eduref.org/Virtual/Lessons/Guide.shtml

For more information on Fishbone diagrams and Gantt charts

www.vertex42.com/ExcelTemplates/fishbone-diagram.html
www.brighthub.com/office/project-management/articles/6179.aspx
www.ganttchart.com/
www.vertex42.com/ExcelTemplates/excel-gantt-chart.html

For more information on the Bologna Declaration

http://ec.europa.eu/education/policies/educ/bologna/bologna.pdf

3

Teaching strategies and approaches to learning

Billy Futter

There are many ways to create learning opportunities for students. For example, through a lecture, discussion group or laboratory practical, or via distance learning or elearning. Courses usually rely on a mix of strategies. The challenge faced by new teachers is to select the best combination of approaches in order to achieve the course outcomes.

This chapter introduces you to a variety of teaching and learning approaches and includes some short exercises to help you feel confident enough to select and design various instructional methods that will optimise the learning of your students.

The intention of this chapter is not to provide an in-depth view of each strategy, but to equip you with enough insight and confidence to deliver a range of learning opportunities. The Resources section at the end of the chapter will direct you to information in greater detail. Regularly accessing these resources for advice and guidance will help you improve your teaching practice.

Who gets credit for good results?

When students achieve outstanding results, it is natural for the teacher to take some of the credit. However, when students fail, the tendency is to blame them for being unmotivated, disinterested or unprepared. It would take a very honest teacher to admit that the blame for failure lay at his or her feet. Even less likely is an acknowledgement that students have succeeded despite, rather than because of, the best efforts of the teacher.

All professionals are expected to accept responsibility for the outcome of their interventions. Teachers are professional educators. This professional commitment is at the heart of managing teaching and learning. It means that the teacher becomes accountable for achieving the educational goals of the students. This **learner-focused approach** emphasises what the learner will be able to do *after* experiencing the learning programme.

Personal view 3.1

At his farewell function, a popular professor at my university attributed the success of his students to the fact that he was a bad lecturer. He explained: 'After each lecture they had to return to the textbook to make sense of what they had just heard.'

Billy, pharmacist

This is very different from the traditional focus on what the teacher is going to do. Critics say that you cannot force the learner to work, concentrate, learn, or be enthusiastic. That may be true, but the way in which you design, deliver and monitor your teaching will have a direct bearing on what the learner does or does not do. And, ultimately, this will influence the extent to which you will be perceived to be a professional teacher as opposed to a disinterested technical expert.

Educational perspectives

There have been many innovations in teaching strategies. Underpinning these strategies is a range of perspectives and concepts that give direction to the way we teach. Boxes 3.1 and 3.2 contain some teaching and learning concepts that you may come across during your time as a teacher.

The success of these concepts usually requires that they are integrated into the overall teaching strategy of the department and that all those involved (both colleagues and students) need to understand what is required. However, innovation entails change and not everyone believes that change is good or necessary.

Teaching methods

When deciding on the best teaching method, consider the number of students in the class, the learning outcomes the students should achieve, and the different learning styles (discussed in Chapter 2). Each teaching method has a group of students who will really benefit from it. However, there will be other students who will be bored or confused. Therefore, a teaching strategy that appeals to all learning styles is likely to be the most effective.

A traditional way of teaching in a university is to deliver a lecture. Other teaching methods include tutorials, workshops, laboratory practicals and research projects. There are advantages and drawbacks to all methods, and each approach requires particular ways of delivering teaching material. Whether you have been asked to give a lecture or lead a workshop you will find some useful tips below.

Box 3.1 Learning concepts

- **Deep** and **surface learning** – the difference between deep insight as opposed to superficial learning (see Chapter 2).
- **Cooperative learning** – students work as a team as opposed to competing as individuals. It is based on group work and requires specific methods to facilitate the success of the group.
- **Active learning** – a learning process centred on the need to solve a real problem that involves action, reflection and personal development.
- **Distance learning** – access to learning when the source of information and the students are separated by time and/or distance. The aim is to deliver a learning experience equivalent to that delivered to students who are physically present.
- **eLearning** (electronic learning) – this refers to the use of electronic technology and resources to enhance teaching and learning.
- **Blended learning** – combining the best of face-to-face and elearning. Examples of blended learning include combinations of classroom instruction, online discussions, group activities and reflective journal tasks.
- **Problem-based/case-based learning** (PBL/CBL) – a teaching strategy where students are presented with a problem and are required to find a meaningful solution.

Lecturing

What do you remember about your own lecture experiences? (see Exercise 3.1).

Lecturing is widely used for several good reasons. Firstly, it is an efficient way of presenting information to lots of people. It is also simple and requires little equipment. Moreover, the same lecture can be delivered more than once.

However, despite being the most commonly used teaching method, lectures are also the most widely criticised of all teaching methods (Gibbs 1981) for the following reasons:

- *Learning style:* Most students are not auditory learners and are easily distracted. Consequently, they forget much of what they have heard.
- *Attention span:* After the first ten minutes of a lecture, the attention span diminishes. It is followed by fidgeting, trance and sometimes sleep!

Box 3.2 Teaching concepts

- **Teaching strategy** – the combination of teaching and learning methods that are used to achieve desired educational outcomes.
- **Educational objectives** – what the teacher aims to achieve.
- **Learning outcomes** – what the student should be able to demonstrate after completing the learning programme. This is verified through assessment.
- **Competencies** – the combination of knowledge, attitudes and skills that make up learning outcomes.
- **Notional hours** – an estimate of the amount of time it will take for the learner to achieve the targeted level of competence. It consists of both the contact time with the teacher and the time spent on independent learning activities (i.e. time for knowledge instruction by the teacher and construction by the student)
- **Social networking** – a process of creating communities of people with similar interests. It is an exploding social phenomenon among the younger generation. Educationalists are increasingly recognising the importance of integrating social networking into their teaching programmes. Examples include Facebook, MySpace and Twitter.

The result may be confusion, boredom, and increasing difficulty in assimilation.

- Lectures tend to promote surface learning and do not include **active learning** tasks, which are better at encouraging reasoning, positive attitudes, motivation to learn and competence.
- Students learn and comprehend at different paces. However, the lecture is presented at the lecturer's pace. Inevitably, the pace will be too fast or too slow for some students.
- One-way communication and large class numbers inhibit questions from students. Misconceptions, incorrect understanding and knowledge gaps may not be identified and corrected.

However, there are several ways in which you can overcome these problems in order to deliver an exciting and engaging lecture.

Top tips for lecture planning

- Make sure your lecture has three parts: an *introduction* to describe the context, what you propose to do, and what you expect of the students; the *body*, which contains the content of the material in a logical sequence; and a *conclusion* to summarise the major points.

- Carve the lecture body into small 'concept' blocks – between five and nine key points. Plan a mini summary to transition between each block.
- Organise the points you want to make, using one or more of the following techniques: use chronological or ascending/descending order; present a problem followed by possible solutions; ask a question followed by short answers and explanations; move from the simple to complex, from familiar to unfamiliar.
- Select meaningful examples to help with understanding and remembering information.
- What is your 'take-home message', that is, what do you expect the students to know at the end of the lecture? Does the lecture material achieve this?
- Budget time for impromptu questions and discussions during the lecture.
- Design ways that will ensure that students interact with the reading material.
- Plan ways to check students' comprehension and competence. Write your examination questions in advance of the lecture and test them during the lecture.

Top tips for lecture delivery

- Before your lecture, check the venue. Ensure that the room is comfortable both for you as the teacher and for the learners. Also make sure you have all the equipment you might need, such as a white board or internet access, and that they are in good working order. Ensure that you have passwords for any computers, pens for the white board, and so on.
- Give useful directions at the beginning of the class such as whether or not students should take notes, supporting chapters in reference materials, how and when to ask questions, and so on.
- Summarise what happened during the last lecture. If you ask a student to do this, it will give you the chance to clarify misunderstandings or provide positive feedback. Frequent

summaries during the lecture are also useful to reinforce major points.

- Speak at an even pace – not too fast or too slow. Vary the volume and tone of your voice. When presenting new ideas or technical terms, repeat, rephrase, and slow down. Pause for emphasis.
- Do not underestimate your non-verbal behaviour. It creates opportunities for the audience to feel and see your enthusiasm. How you use your arms and hands helps to convey emphasis and visual meaning. Make eye contact with the students – looking at the audience will give you clues about levels of boredom, inability to hear you, or lack of understanding. If you are nervous you may find the tips in Box 3.3 useful.
- Move around the room. Contrary to what some lecturers believe, the lectern is neither a life raft nor a protective screen. It does not save you from the audience. If you cling to it too tightly, your bloodless fingers will show! Reduce the space between you and the audience to personalise the communication and to make it more comfortable for them to answer questions in front of the whole class.
- Follow your lecture plan but allow for spontaneity.
- Do not read from notes or a book for an extended length of time. Use visual aids to illustrate and provide structure to the lecture, not as a tool to prompt your memory.
- Keep your audience interested. Adapt material to their beliefs, values and priorities. Introduce a relevant current controversy to spark interest in the topic. Use humour, but not at the students' expense. Be enthusiastic – you don't have to be an entertainer but you should be excited by your topic. Do something different every 15 to 25 minutes – such as pose a question, put up a new slide, or break into small groups.

Spicing up lectures

You can also incorporate other teaching methods into lectures to improve their effectiveness.

Discussions

Instead of you doing all the talking, why not try introducing some discussion time into your lecture?

Whole group discussions can be very effective when used in conjunction with other teaching methods. They provide for greater interaction

Box 3.3 Overcoming nerves

It is natural to feel tension before standing up in front of a large group of people for the first time. The key is to build your confidence. This is derived from good preparation, rehearsal, using key words as prompts, breaking up the presentation into digestible chunks, and being confident in the use of visual aids. In other words, eliminate any variable that you are not sure about.

Think of it as hosting a dinner party – dress appropriately, arrive before the guests, welcome the guests, provide a small but interesting starter, a nice blend of three or four items for the main course (suitably presented and easily digestible), and a tasty sweet as a memorable conclusion.

Plan an ice-breaker to get the guests talking to each other, do not dominate the conversation, and use humour sparingly and appropriately.

between the lecturer and students, and help build relationships. The lecturer maintains control over the learning topic by steering the discussion. The possibility of being called upon to answer questions also tends to increase student focus during a lecture.

You could ask students to reflect on their experiences relating to the subject of the lecture or perhaps challenge their knowledge and values with provocative questions. You can also try asking them about the meaning or relevance of the material. If you expect students to engage with, and apply, theoretical concepts, they may benefit from readings and discussion topics in advance of the lecture.

The discussion process requires some planning and control to prevent it from getting out of hand. Students who have weak note-taking skills may find it difficult to grasp key points during the discussion. In this case, it may be helpful if you reiterate these after the discussion.

Another stumbling block is that some students will be too intimidated to take part in discussions, particularly in front of the whole class. Bear in mind that the thought of being picked to contribute may leave some students preferring not to come to your lecture rather than having their name called out in front of the class! However, there are some techniques you can use to reduce students' apprehension:

- Build their confidence slowly. More students are likely to respond if they are first given the opportunity to engage in small group discussions (five or six people) or discussions with their neighbours.

- Reduce the physical space between you and the students – walk up the aisle or between rows of seats so that students do not have to shout across a large lecture theatre.
- Paraphrase the student's response. You can usually make it sound more effective than the student. This also allows the rest of the class to hear and understand what the volunteer has said.
- Provide positive feedback for their participation, either in front of the class and/or individually after the class.

Guest speakers

Inviting a speaker to talk during your lecture is a refreshing change for both you and your students. They can share experiences and provide an alternative point of view. Patients, alternative therapists, clinicians, hospital administrators or insurers make excellent guest speakers and can provide insight relevant to the students.

If your guest is not comfortable talking for a length of time in front of the class invite her or him to take part in a question and answer session. This gives you control over the presentation and you will be able to direct the session to cover areas that are particularly interesting to the students and that expose them to specific learning opportunities. You could also invite students to ask questions or offer opinions at appropriate times.

The guest speaker session will be more effective if the students have insight into the topics that will be covered. If the topic has not been covered in advance, make sure that there is *interesting* prescribed reading.

Case studies

One major challenge with teaching is to create learning opportunities that move the students from 'know' to 'know how', and from 'show' to 'show how'. **Case studies** serve this purpose. Also known as simulations, their purpose is to demonstrate theoretical concepts in an applied setting, and to reflect reality. In a case study, students are required to produce solutions to problems identified in a real-world situation. The case is carefully designed to raise the key issues desired by the lecturer.

Case studies help to bridge the gap between theory and practice, and encourage active learning. They also give the students an opportunity for trial and error without the serious consequences from failure in a real world setting. They are useful for creating learning opportunities when there are complex, integrated issues or difficult concepts such as ethical issues (Edinger *et al.* 1999).

Depending upon how they are used, case studies also provide an opportunity to develop transferable skills such as working in teams, gathering information and analysis, time management, presentation skills and problem solving. Case studies have been shown to increase students' enjoyment of the topic and their desire to learn. They have the added bonus that teachers who have used them also find the process enjoyable.

There are different ways to use a case study:

- The teacher presents the case. This can be on paper, or as a verbal presentation, and could be illustrated with the use of PowerPoint slides or videos.
- Students role-play the case, having been given the script in advance. The class comments on the role-play and students can reflect on their experience.
- Real patients can be invited to describe their own experiences. Their personal stories make strong impressions on students. Small groups of students can analyse the case and develop solutions for the problems reported.
- Trained, patient actors act out the case with the students.
- Computer-generated simulated patients are increasingly popular because of their flexible use and ease with which they can be repeated. See Resources at the end of the chapter for more information.

Small group teaching

Stimulating learning is often more effective when dealing with fewer students. Working with small groups also facilitates the development of a professional relationship between the teacher and the class, a critical feature of all successful professional interactions (Futter 2009a). In addition, small groups help to build the interpersonal skills of students, skills that are increasingly recognised as important to develop in students and health professionals.

When working with small groups of students, your role will be more like that of a facilitator than a teacher. A facilitator's job is to ensure that both the task is achieved and the group functioning is maintained. A good facilitator will:

- Create a comfortable learning environment for the students
- Motivate students to set goals, measure their own progress and be aware of their development
- Encourage students to feel good about their work
- Provide appropriate learning experiences.

The success of small group learning is very dependent upon the members of the groups. When forming small groups of students, consider getting a mix of characteristics, such as gender, cultures, skills and experiences. The emphasis is on cooperative, rather than competitive, learning (Johnson and Johnson 2011). This is not likely to happen if some group members believe that working in the group will compromise their overall mark, that is, if they gain nothing from interdependence. In addition, the group will not thrive if some members either do not accept their responsibilities or are not held accountable for the group's performance, or if the process allows one person to dominate.

You can maximise the success of small group work by using thee following principles.

- Keep the size of the group small, preferably between five and ten members.
- Include both individual and group assessment.
- Maintain regular contact with groups to observe balanced contributions.
- Assign one student in each group the role of recorder, reporter or leader, depending upon the assignment.
- Ensure that each student has a responsibility for teaching other group members one aspect of the assignment.

Brainstorming

The technique of brainstorming is used to generate a variety of opinions. The emphasis is to stimulate creativity. The principles used to encourage contributions and minimise social inhibitions are:

- Do not criticise.
- Generate quantity – the more ideas, the better the chance of finding the best solution.
- Praise unusual ideas – this will encourage students to think creatively.
- Combine ideas rather than seek a single solution.

Brainstorming is often used in team building and can generate fun and enthusiasm (see Resources at the end of the chapter for more information).

Tutorials

A tutorial is a regular meeting of a small group of students in which the tutor facilitates the learning process. Usually this is once a week for about an hour. At these meetings the learners present solutions to problems that have been set in advance. One-on-one tutoring is also an option but is more difficult to build into a formal learning programme.

Learners are expected to assume responsibility for their academic challenges, as facilitated by the tutor. Although tutors have a responsibility for explaining, guiding, teaching and correcting their tutees, their primary function is to listen and ask questions more than to provide answers.

Extensive preparation is usually required before the tutorial. Students should spend a considerable amount of time reading, writing, researching, solving problems, or developing experimental technique.

It is helpful to students to provide them with a written statement detailing the expectations for the work to be accomplished during tutorials, and a description of how they will be evaluated. Your university may have its own specific policies and procedures for conducting these sessions.

If you are going to use tutorials in the learning programme, make sure that you have trained tutors. You may find it useful to ask them to complete an online tutor training course (see Resources at end of chapter).

A successful tutor:

- Sets the agenda
- Has a relaxed interaction with the students, a sense of humour and the ability to 'lighten up' a situation
- Gets to know their students' strengths and weaknesses and works through the strengths to improve the weaknesses
- Shows empathy with problems and makes students feel good about themselves and what they have achieved
- Ends the session on a positive note.

Mentoring

Mentoring is about developing people. It is a strategy that can be used in many different situations. In simple terms, mentoring is a process in which a more experienced person supports and guides a less-experienced person in his or her personal or professional development.

The foundation is a trusting relationship that is characterised by care and empathy. In this relationship, the mentor becomes a friend, an adviser, a guide and a role model. They support, challenge and provide vision for their mentees. This helps the mentee to 'learn the ropes', take on greater responsibility and become a more mature, confident person. In a nutshell, mentors help their mentees to help themselves.

Having a mentor can make a big difference for professionals who are transitioning into new roles. It is also invaluable for students entering unfamiliar environments in which they are unsure what is expected of them (for example, when starting their first year at university, clinical rotations and community placements).

Mentoring is distinct from tutoring; a tutor helps students come to terms with teaching material, whereas a mentor is a personal facilitator who empowers mentees to achieve certain goals and cope with the learning environment.

A mentoring programme has many benefits for both mentors and mentees, both individually and as a group. It requires:

- A clear statement of programme purpose and goals
- A recruitment and selection plan for mentors
- A support and training programme for mentors
- A monitoring and evaluation process for the programme.

Personal view 3.2

Over the years I have developed and refined a group research project which not only introduces students to conducting research but also substantially improves their communication and interpersonal skills.

Groups of five students are expected to conduct and present research on public health issues. They are required to evaluate an educational intervention in an area where they had identified an information deficit. They design questionnaires, prepare a patient information leaflet, conduct interviews, prepare a written research report, develop a web page and a poster, and give a verbal presentation of the project.

The students also develop interpersonal and leadership skills by learning how to identify and respond to different social styles. Within the group they agree on group norms and standards, conflict resolution processes, rewards and penalties.

Each group forms a business unit with a name, a budget, and a mission statement.

Assessment of the project includes students' reflection on the development of their new skills as well as on the research.

Joseph, senior clinical lecturer

A successful mentoring programme will result in the development of a support network among the students. Both mentors and mentees experience increased motivation, self-confidence and personal growth.

Research projects

Designing research projects for small groups of students is an excellent opportunity to achieve a variety of learning objectives through integrating various course components (see Personal view 3.2). It provides a learning context that is of interest to the students, especially if they are allowed to select their own topics.

Communication, negotiation and management skills are developed, as well as cooperative learning between group members.

Workshops

A workshop is an effective way to stimulate discussion, create alternative solutions to problems and develop action points.

For the workshop you will need to lay out tables and chairs in groups and ensure you have enough materials for each group. Useful equipment includes flip charts, different coloured marker pens, coloured stickers, and paper and pens for making notes.

As a facilitator of the workshop you will need to explain the agenda, the process of the workshop, and your role as facilitator. It may help to set the scene with a brief presentation that contextualises the issues you wish to cover within the workshop. Clearly identify the reason for the workshop, the questions to be addressed and the time limits for each stage.

When the students are in their groups it is a good idea to suggest an ice breaker to provide an opportunity for them to meet each other. Each group should then assign one member as a group leader to guide discussion and solicit points of view, and a scribe to record the discussion on a flip chart or a computer that can be projected on to a screen for the audience to read.

The groups discuss their mandates for a specified period. When the larger group is reconvened, group leaders present the opinions of their group. As each group reports, their key points are recorded by the scribe for the whole group to see. After each group has reported, the facilitator opens the floor for discussions. Any additional points are also recorded on the flip chart or computer.

The group as a whole can then discuss the outcomes and comment on action points. As a facilitator you should summarise the outcomes and action points of the session.

Laboratory practicals

Teaching through the use of practicals may contribute a significant proportion of the taught component of the curriculum. It also accounts for the majority of one-on-one contact time with students.

Why practicals?

Practicals are based on the concept of experiential learning in which students learn by carrying out tasks and critically evaluating the outcomes of the task, identifying problems, and proposing improvements.

Aims of practicals

These usually consist of the following:

- Linking and reinforcing theory with practice
- Learning how to use equipment and developing hands-on skills and techniques
- Improving understanding of scientific methods through their practical application
- Conducting scientific research such as method design, data collection and analysis, presenting findings
- Developing professional skills, such as developing problem solving and critical thinking skills; developing an appreciation for and the skill of

working accurately and efficiently; working both independently and as part of a team; assertiveness

- Providing opportunities for staff and student contact to discuss the subject
- Providing a setting in which staff can observe the progress of individual students and intervene if necessary.

For the first few years, students are usually required to follow protocols. Later they might be challenged to take responsibility for designing their own experiments and, ultimately, undertake advanced postgraduate research.

The teaching team

Practical sessions usually run for several hours. They are supervised by academic staff, laboratory technicians and trained demonstrators who may be undergraduate or postgraduate students. This team is responsible for the effective and safe study of the learners.

Health and safety

Health and safety are critical issues in practicals. Check the policies and procedures in place to minimise risk in each practical at your institution.

Each member of the teaching team will have specific responsibilities, but if you are the person in charge, you have overall responsibility to ensure compliance with the institution codes of practice and relevant legislation.

Check where the nearest trained first-aider is and be familiar with the procedures for responding to and recording accidents.

Hints, tips and suggestions

Organising practical work is time-consuming and should be started early. Ensure that supplies are ordered and that equipment is organised and checked. Work closely with the technical team responsible for the teaching laboratories and equipment.

Demonstrators contribute significantly to the success of practicals, but you should make sure that they are fully briefed. If necessary, organise training sessions for them so that they can carry out all the procedures and techniques with confidence and can respond to questions appropriately and effectively.

Consider assessment issues when designing the practicals: should practical reports be graded, and if so, how? To what extent should these marks form a component of the formative and summative assessment of the course? (See Chapter 4 for more information on assessment.)

Think about the progression of skills across the years of the degree programme: the skills the students are bringing to your practical/laboratory class; what they are gaining from the class; and the skills they will need in future practical/project work.

Laboratories for clinical skills

The shift in emphasis to the clinical role of healthcare professionals has not undermined the value of laboratory work. However, laboratory work has moved away from repetitive technical skills and now tends to focus on responding to patient scenarios presented in the form of case studies. The ideal clinical laboratory course would involve computer-generated simulated patients. Most programmes have detailed set-up instructions and user-friendly features for saving, analysing, and reporting results. Students are able to process and analyse the signals both in real-time and later offline.

The professional environment

Most training institutions expect healthcare students to undertake work experience in a professional environment, either in their own time or as part of the academic programme. The effectiveness of this experience is substantially improved through the integration of specific learning tasks to be performed during placement. For example, ask the student to find the package insert for a particular medicine and identify its serious side-effects. They can record the data they find in a book, and reflect on how they would communicate these to a patient. They could also ask the pharmacist in charge whether any patients have mentioned these problems.

The difficulty of these tasks increases as the students progress in their academic careers. The tasks are designed with a specific purpose – to equip the student with the professional and scientific awareness required for the next phase of their training.

A big challenge that has been grossly underestimated by those increasing the clinical component of the curriculum is the need for competent supervisors, or **preceptors** (ASCP 2011). Clinical encounters lose much of their value without a preceptor showing students the way, asking them challenging questions, providing them with support and defending them should the need arise.

Effective preceptors are passionate about their work and are able to immerse their students in the learning situation, allowing them to gain new knowledge from their peers and the environment. They stimulate the imagination, and keep students hooked on the experience.

Experiential learning should always be accompanied by specific tasks, guidelines, reflection and feedback, regardless of where the experience takes place.

Self-directed learning

Seamless education throughout a professional career underpins the concept of **self-directed learning** (SDL). As its name implies, this approach to learning emphasises that learners have some responsibility for their own learning. Learners – particularly in the early stages of their development – need to develop this skill, ideally with facilitation from a teacher, supervisor or mentor.

The importance of developing student capacity for SDL cannot be over-estimated. A commitment to lifelong learning is non-negotiable for health professionals. Professional success will depend on learners developing the ability to design and implement continuing professional development (CPD) opportunities to elevate and update their competencies. SDL facilitates this development as well as producing autonomous practitioners who can learn for themselves.

SDL challenges the notion that everything must be taught by someone else, and also brings workplace learning to life. But this does not mean that learning is no longer the responsibility of the teacher. In fact, the reverse is true – the teacher is accountable for creating the environment in which the student is confident to accept this role and demonstrate professional competence.

A practical definition of SDL (Jubraj 2009) is that it is about health professionals being personally responsible for attaining the required competencies in the workplace in order to achieve fitness to practise, supported by the infrastructure of an accredited training centre or other designated organisation.

While this method of learning makes sense for senior practitioners who can identify their own learning and development needs, SDL has attracted some controversy in situations where newly qualified practitioners are expected to make clinical decisions. To the extent that they are 'unconsciously incompetent' (see Chapter 6), patient safety demands that their learning be guided and supported. Under these circumstances it is sometimes appropriate to teach junior practitioners in situations where they don't know what they don't know; but it is also possible to inspire a sense of SDL through:

1 Listening and asking questions where possible rather than persistently telling or advising
2 Facilitating junior practitioners to identify problems and what it is they need or want to learn
3 Giving feedback on performance rapidly, regularly and effectively.

Top tips for appropriate use of SDL

- Define SDL in your own learning context to clarify expectations of learners and other practitioners.
- Agree what needs to be learned by your students, mindful of whether they are bound by a curriculum or are qualified practitioners providing patient care.

- Encourage the student to be self-directed in how they learn, providing facilitation as necessary.
- Avoid sending the student away to read a textbook or journal without any form of follow-up.
- Remember that SDL covers individual instances of learning as well as how the student manages their overall learning.
- Align expectations and responsibilities between yourself and your students (see Box 3.4).

Box 3.4 *Learning contracts*

A learning contract is a formal agreement written by a learner. It details what will be learned, how the learning will be achieved, measurable indicators of progress, and the specific evaluation criteria to be used in judging the completion of the learning. It specifies the learner's expectations of the teacher and what they feel the lecturer could reasonably expect from the learner. Treat this is as formal document, signed by both learner and teacher. Review performance regularly.

Sample learning contracts can be placed on a web page for learners to use as an example. Even better, encourage them to use the discussion forum to brainstorm ideas for the design of a standard class learning contract. Learning contracts clarify expectations and help the teacher and learner share the responsibility for learning.

---

eLearning

Developments in information and communication technology (ICT) have had a huge influence on teaching and learning. The most obvious impact has been on distance learning. However, it has also led to a combination of face-to-face and online instruction known as **blended learning** or hybrid learning. These innovations have been widely adopted in healthcare training institutions.

eLearning is characterised by being facilitated by teaching staff, integrated into the overall teaching and learning programme, and distributed using electronic media. Other terms you may come across include:

1 *Web based instruction/learning* – teaching delivered via the web, available on-demand.

2 *Distributed virtual instruction* – learning occurs through the use of technologies when teacher and learner are physically distant.

3 *Information and communications technology (ICT)/Electronic-based instructional resources (EBIR)/Computer-aided learning (CAL)* – these are all terms that describe the medium used to teach.

4 *Online classrooms/virtual classrooms/learning networks* – where the learning takes place.

5 **Distance learning** – education delivered to students who are not physically present.

eLearning is significantly different from traditional classroom teaching. For example, students are no longer completely dependent on faculty members as the primary source of knowledge. Teaching strategies have changed from information transfer to collaborative, active and guided learning. This has coincided with the development of a variety of web-based systems to facilitate teaching, learning and assessment.

Learning management systems

Learning management systems (LMSs) or virtual learning environments (VLEs) have evolved to enable teachers to design and deliver courses by making resources available online and by engaging students in online activities. *Moodle* (an open source software) and *Blackboard* (a commercial software) are two of the most popular LMSs used globally. These systems are designed to create a virtual learning environment in which one can use a variety of online instructional strategies. In other words, they cater for a full range of interactive teaching methods.

Some of the typical LMS options available to those designing elearning courses are:

- Storing files (e.g. lecture notes, presentations, submission of assignments by students)
- Linking to additional resources such as web sites, additional reading, videos
- Creating discussion groups (e.g. to debate controversial issues, to post research findings for the class to review)
- Use of student journals/diaries for reflective writing with opportunity for feedback from teaching staff
- Employing small group teaching as a strategy to encourage active participation by each student
- Using a variety of formative and summative assessment options, for example, submission of assignments, peer assessment and MCQs
- Use of surveys (e.g. canvassing student opinion about a topic or ongoing course evaluations for continuous quality improvement)

- Creating web sites, wikis and blogs that allow students to move from being consumers to being creators of web-based information.

Preparation

Detailed planning is needed before launching an elearning course. Although most of the different options are relatively easy to set up, facilitation of learning, such as online forums, is time consuming. There is a very real danger of overloading both learners and teachers, and becoming so overwhelmed with technical issues that you will run out of time to stimulate discussion and provide adequate feedback. This would severely affect the success of your teaching innovations. The best advice is to seek guidance from a technology expert at your institution or someone experienced in using elearning strategies.

The value of elearning

The revolution in information technology has made vast amounts of educational resources easily accessible. In addition, the Open Educational Resources (OER) movement aims to make such high-quality resources available free of charge. Research in higher education has shown that elearning can:

- Improve student performance
- Increase access, allowing students to attend courses across physical, political, economic and time boundaries, and usually at lower cost
- Provide highly valued convenience and flexibility to learners: in many contexts, elearning is self-paced and the learning sessions are available 24 hours a day, seven days a week
- Help students to develop the digital literacy skills required in their discipline, profession or career.

What future is there for elearning?

Developments in communication technology have been widely embraced by the global community, especially by the younger generation. The marriage of these innovations has opened the door for major changes in teaching and learning. Significant changes are forecast in the near future, especially with the emphasis on social networks, and the developments that have taken place with cell phone technology.

What computer games could help to facilitate the learning of your students? How could you use social networking sites such as Facebook, Twitter or MySpace to create a strong social, professional and learning network that will help to support the development of cultural competence?

How can I easily introduce elearning as a teaching strategy?

When using elearning strategies, the interaction between teacher and student changes dramatically. Teachers who are accustomed to the traditional classroom learning environment will need to adapt their teaching methods and materials in response to this new setting.

The following are examples of instructional strategies that have been used successfully in the traditional classroom and can be used very effectively with elearning.

Lecture

It is possible to present online lectures in many different ways. These include a combination of lecture notes, PowerPoint presentations, and audio or video presentations. The option also exists to create links to other virtual resources. LMS lectures are typically shorter than the traditional presentations. They are more focused and provide enough information to serve as a basis for further reading or other learning activities.

Mentoring

The main benefit for setting up an LMS mentoring system is the opportunity for frequent and convenient communication between mentor and student.

Small group learning

LMSs are ideally suited for using a variety of small group formats. For example, group projects can include discussion groups, role-play, simulations, group collaborative work, debates, brainstorming and games. Students are able to discuss content, share ideas and solve problems at times convenient to themselves, with resources readily available. Factors such as geography, gender or disabilities do not disadvantage students in this environment.

Collaborative learning

Collaborative learning is the process of getting two or more students to work together to achieve learning outcomes. Online learning models are natural environments for collaborative learning, but they are not collaborative learning environments by definition. Learning activities should be specifically and carefully designed in order to work effectively.

Forums

A forum is an open discussion conducted by one or more resource persons (e.g. a knowledgeable invited guest) and an entire group. As the lecturer you will moderate and guide the discussion and encourage the students to raise and discuss issues, present alternative opinions, offer information, or ask questions of the resource person(s).

An online forum can be more effective than the lecture theatre. Members of a discussion panel, experts and the moderator can take part without having to travel or be available at a particular time. Unlike face-to-face discussions in large lecture theatres, participating in an online forum provides students (and teachers) with space to consider contributions carefully before posting them. This is particularly useful for shy students who lack confidence or students who have a different mother tongue from the language of instruction.

Summary

Classrooms, lecture theatres, laboratories, professional settings and online environments each influence the way we teach. Some teaching strategies will suit particular environments better than others and will more effectively meet the course objectives. However, the ways in which we utilise the strategies will differ as we make the best use of the characteristics and capacities of each environment.

Remember that students tend to learn what they want to know and remember what they understand. Your teaching strategy should ensure that the knowledge has a context that is familiar to the students and facilitates their understanding.

Top tips

- Create a favourable and comfortable learning environment.
- Accept criticism and be prepared to change.
- Plan carefully but be flexible.
- Things do go wrong, especially technical equipment, and sometimes your memory – apologise, adapt and move on.
- Show passion and commitment, both to the subject and to the learners. Nothing else makes a bigger difference between a tedious and an enjoyable learning experience.

Exercise 3.1 Your lecture experiences

Think back on your experiences with lectures – those in which you fell asleep and those that left you invigorated. Picture your positive and negative role models. Why were they so good or bad? This should help you to compile a very personal list of what worked and what failed dismally.

References and further reading

ASCP (2011). *Become a Preceptor*. Alexandria, VA: American Society of Consultant Pharmacists. http://www.ascp.com/articles/become-preceptor (accessed 11 March 2011).

Austin Z *et al*. (2006). Simulated patients vs. standardized patients in objective structured clinical examinations. *American Journal of Pharmaceutical Education* October 15; 70(5): 119. www.ncbi.nlm.nih.gov/pmc/articles/PMC1636998/ (accessed 26 February 2011).

Beck DE. Clinical simulations: their curricular role now and in the future. In: *OSCES and Virtual Patient Simulations in Pharmacy Education: International Experiences and Research Findings*. Alexandria, VA: American Association of Colleges of Pharmacy. www.aacp.org/meetingsandevents/AM/Documents/Annual%20Meeting%202008/Tuesday/OSCEsVirtualPatients.pdf (accessed 26 February 2011).

Edinger W *et al*. (1999). Using standardized patients to teach clinical ethics. *Med Educ Online* [serial online] 4(6). www.med-ed-online.org/t0000010.htm (accessed 26 February 2011).

Florin L, Sugioka S (May 2007). *Teachers as learners and learners as teachers*. Edited by Patti Horne. http://en.wikibooks.org/wiki/Change_Issues_in_Curriculum_and_Instruction/The_Teacher_as_Learner_and_the_Learner_as_Teacher (accessed 26 February 2011).

Futter B (2007). *Culture, Professionalism and the Practice of Pharmacy*. Presented at FIP International Conference, Beijing, China, September 2007. www.slideshare.net/billy.futter/culture-professionalism-and-the-practice-of-pharmacy#stats-bottom (accessed 26 February 2011).

Futter B (2009a). Improving performance by working with others. Building trust – the defining factor: Part 1 What and why? *South African Pharmaceutical Journal* September: 48–49. www.sapj.co.za/index.php/SAPJ/article/viewFile/665/609 (accessed 23 March 2011).

Gibbs G (1981). Twenty terrible reasons for lecturing. *SCED Occasional Paper No. 8* Birmingham. 1981. Available from Oxford Centre for staff and learning development. www.brookes.ac.uk/services/ocsd/2_learntch/20reasons.html (accessed 26 February 2011).

Heppner F (2007). *Teaching the Large College Class: A Guidebook for Instructors with Multitudes*. San Francisco, CA: Jossey-Bass.

James D *et al*. (December 2001). The design and evaluation of a simulated-patient teaching programme to develop the consultation skills of undergraduate pharmacy students. *Pharmacy World and Science* 23(6): 212–216. www.springerlink.com/content/bppg0lq9c9mhxl8p/.

Johnson DW, Johnson RT (2011). *An Overview of Cooperative Learning*. Edina, MN: Cooperative Learning Institute. http://www.co-operation.org/ (accessed 11 March 2011).

Jubraj B (2009). Developing a culture of self-directed workplace learning in pharmacy. *The Pharmaceutical Journal* 283: 47–48.

A brief guide to notional hours

https://www.ru.ac.za/documents/Institutional%20Planning/Brief%20Guide%20to%20%20Credits%20&%20Notional%20Hours.pdf.

A guide to the role of social networking in education

www.slideshare.net/acarvin/social-networking-and-education.

More information on cooperative, active and problem-based learning

www.co-operation.org/.

https://www.ru.ac.za/documents/Institutional%20Planning/Brief%20Guide%20to%20%20Credits%20&%20Notional%20Hours.pdf.

www.udel.edu/inst/.

Rhem J (1998). Problem-based learning: an introduction. *The National Teaching & Learning FORUM* 8(1). www.ntlf.com/html/pi/9812/pbl_1.htm (accessed 22 March 2010).

Ways to improve the use of visual aids and presentations

www.slideshare.net/thecroaker/death-by-powerpoint.
www.slideshare.net/jhaustin/presentation-tips.

Using case studies to teach clinical ethics

Edinger W *et al*. (1999). Using standardized patients to teach clinical ethics. *Med Educ Online* [serial online] 4(6). www.med-ed-online.org/t0000010.htm.

More information on patient simulations

Marriott JL (2007). Development and implementation of a computer-generated 'virtual' patient program. *Pharmacy Education* 7(4): 335–340.

Marriott JL (2007). Use and evaluation of 'virtual' patients for assessment of clinical pharmacy undergraduates. *Pharmacy Education* 7(4): 341–349.

Mesquita A *et al*. (2010). Developing communication skills in pharmacy: A systematic review of the use of simulated patient methods. *Patient Education and Counseling* 78(2): 143–148. linkinghub.elsevier.com/retrieve/pii/S0738399109003139 (accessed 26 February 2011).

Thompson JE (1994). Development and use of an interactive database management system for simulated patient care experiences for pharmacy students. *American Journal of Pharmaceutical Education* 58: 324–332. www.ajpe.org/legacy/pdfs/aj5803324.pdf (accessed 26 February 2011).

Teaching small groups

Futter B (2009b). Improving performance by working with others. Building trust – the defining factor: Part 1 What and why? *SA Pharmaceutical Journal* **76**(8). www.sapj.co.za/index.php/SAPJ/article/viewFile/665/609 (accessed 26 February 2011).

Futter B (2009c). Improve performance by working with others: Trust – the defining factor: Part 2: How? *SA Pharmaceutical Journal* **76**(10). www.sapj.co.za/index.php/SAPJ/article/view/714/650 (accessed 26 February 2011).

Gerber RE (2011). *Facilitation Skills for Effective, Active Learning*. South Africa: Port Elizabeth Technikon. http://www.nmmu.ac.za/robert/facilitation/Default.htm (accessed 23 March 2011).

Honors Tutorial College (2006). *What is a Tutorial?* Athens, OH: Ohio University. www.honors.ohio.edu/tutorial.htm (accessed 26 February 2011).

Small Group Instructor Training Course (SGITC) Student Reference, June 1998. Chapter 6: *Small Group Instruction: Theory and Practice*. http://www.au.af.mil/au/awc/awcgate/sgitc/read6.htm (accessed 14 March 2011).

More information on brainstorming

http://en.wikipedia.org/wiki/Brainstorming.

Help with tutor training

LERN 10 – Online Tutor Training Project. http://www.ccsf.edu/Services/LAC/Lern10_Online_Tutor_Training/ (accessed 14 March).

Lynchburg College (2011). *Tutoring Strategies*. Lynchburg, VA: Lynchburg College. www.lynchburg.edu/x2377.xml (accessed 26 February 2011).

Help with designing a mentoring programme

MENTOR (2009). *Elements of Effective Practice for Mentoring.* Alexandria, VA: National Mentoring Partnership. http://www.mentoring.org/downloads/mentoring_1222.pdf (accessed 12 March 2011).
Office of Faculty and Organizational Development (2011). *Faculty Mentoring.* East Lansing, MI: Michigan State University. http://fod.msu.edu/LeadershipResources/mentoring/index.asp#3 (accessed 26 February 2011).

How to develop a laboratory programme

Capehart KD (2008). A laboratory exercise in capsule making. *American Journal of Pharmaceutical Education* **72**(5).
Sobieraj DM *et al.* (2009). Redesign and evaluation of a patient assessment course. *American Journal of Pharmaceutical Education* **73**(7). www.ajpe.org/view.asp?art=aj7307133& pdf=yes (accessed 26 February 2011).

Help on how to run workshops

www.businessballs.com/workshops.htm.

A guide to precepting

ASCP (2011). *Become a Preceptor.* Alexandria, VA: American Society of Consultant Pharmacists. http://www.ascp.com/articles/become-preceptor (accessed 11 March 2011).

More on self-directed learning

Jubraj B (2009). Developing a culture of self-directed workplace learning in pharmacy. *The Pharmaceutical Journal* **283**: 47–48.
Mills E, Black P (2009). Self-directed learning and advanced practice development in pharmacy. *The Pharmaceutical Journal* **283**: 535. www.pjonline.com/news/selfdirected_learning_practice_development (accessed 26 February 2011).

More information on eLearning and related useful sites

http://en.wikipedia.org/wiki/E-learning.
http://moodle.org/.
www.jiscinfonet.ac.uk/case-studies/tangible.
www.educause.edu/7Things.
www.jiscinfonet.ac.uk/infokits/index_html.
www.jisc.ac.uk/.

4

Assessing learning

Timothy Rennie

Assessment is an established and often ongoing part of most of our lives. Assessment goes hand in hand with education, training and learning. Therefore, most people have been assessed at some point, and usually from an early age. As a teacher you will inevitably be presented with an opportunity to mark, grade or indicate the level of competence or performance of your students through assessment. The purpose of this chapter is to give you a quick guide to the core principles of assessment and to understand the why, what and how. It also presents a selection of assessment techniques that can be used individually or together in different settings.

What is assessment?

Assessment is often thought of as a way to quantify or qualify previous learning and/or direct future learning. Another way to help define the concept of assessment is by providing examples of how it is conducted.

Methods of assessment can be classified in a number of different ways. In Fig. 4.1 they are categorised as oral, written or practical. You can see from the diagram that there can be a cross-over between these various methods of assessment. For example, the **Objective Structured Clinical Examination** (OSCE – see the appropriate section later in this chapter for more information) usually incorporates oral and written elements as well as practical skills.

Assessment methods may also be described as quantitative or qualitative in nature. For example, a **Multiple Choice Question** (MCQ) is a pre-defined, sometimes pre-validated method and will have pre-defined answers. So structured is the nature of MCQ assessment that they are sometimes marked or graded by automated machines.

Conversely, an oral viva voce examination (meaning 'by word of mouth') will usually be based on the student's dissertation or thesis. While there are guidelines for conducting viva examinations, the examiners will have a large degree of subjective freedom – and necessarily so – to question, probe, discuss and debate. This may relate to information not included in the thesis, such as the decisions made by the learner, and even their

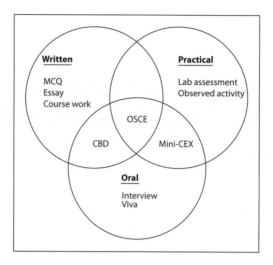

Figure 4.1. Methods of assessment.

motivations or aspirations in conducting their work. The examiners will have no direct control over the responses that the learner delivers and, therefore, the answers cannot be pre-defined.

Formative, summative and ongoing assessment

Most learners experience some degree of **ongoing assessment**, be it a test at the beginning of the class on the previous lesson or structured formal modular examinations throughout a course or degree. The marks may or may not contribute to a final mark – they may just indicate how well you are progressing. They may be used to deliberately motivate learning, or this could just be an unintended side-effect. However, the concept of ongoing assessment does not really capture this motivational element, whether the assessments are intended to inform future learning or simply provide an indication or 'benchmark' for how much learning has happened.

From another way of defining types of assessment is whether they inform learning progression or whether they provide an indication of how much learning has taken place. **Formative assessment** *informs* learning, whereas **summative assessment** is the *sum* of learning.

From this perspective a single assessment method may be used for different purposes. It may be used to indicate how learners are progressing throughout a learning experience (formative) and in this way point to strengths or gaps in knowledge or skills. This in turn can direct the focus of the learner's learning. Conversely, the assessment may be used as an end-point (summative) examination, such as an end-of-year assessment in a degree course. However, in both these examples the assessment can be described as 'ongoing' despite serving different purposes.

There are some examples of assessment tools at the end of this chapter that can provide a comprehensive assessment of an individual's learning over a period of time (see 'Common assessment methods used in health professions education'). To help you decide which method of assessment is most suitable for your learners it is useful to ask yourself these questions:

- Why am I assessing, what is the purpose?
- What am I assessing against?
- Who is being assessed and who is the assessor?
- At what point in the learner's education or development is the assessment taking place?
- In what setting will the assessment be performed?
- How do I judge what is 'good'?
- How do I feed back the results to the learner?

Why assess?

Questioning why we are assessing may lead us to consider the philosophy and ethics of assessment, which we will not go into here. The purpose of this chapter is to outline the pragmatic perspective: understanding the 'why' may inform better the 'how' and the 'what' (see Exercise 4.1).

Assessment is used to demonstrate a level of **competence** (see Box 4.1). This can be particularly important if someone's competence has a profound and direct impact on others (for example, in medical practice). Assessment may also be part of a selection process such as degree entry examinations or interviews for employment. Assessment is also used as a management tool – to provide evidence of incompetence or poor practice, or to demonstrate value and stimulate activity or competition.

There may also be other, more ignoble, motivations for assessment. Assessment could (but should not) be used to catch people out or to deliberately set levels that people cannot attain in order to exclude or demote. This highlights the importance of assessment being valid, practical and fair.

What am I assessing against?

You may already be able to answer the question why you are assessing. The overall aim may be to demonstrate competence or simply to show that learning has occurred. However, it may not be immediately clear what you are assessing against. There may be a general **curriculum** – this will usually give a broad summary of what is expected of learners and, therefore, what should be assessed. Outside the academic setting you are more likely to find competencies – whether defined or not – that are expected to be attained for an individual to carry out their job or role sufficiently.

Box 4.1 Some definitions (UK setting)

Competencies: 'Competencies are descriptors of the performance criteria, knowledge and understanding that are required to undertake work activities. They describe what individuals need to do, and to know, to carry out a particular job role or function, regardless of who performs it.'

(Competence Framework, NHS Connecting for Health)

Assessment: 'The process of measuring an individual's progress and accomplishments against defined standards and criteria, which often includes an attempt at measurement. The purpose of assessment in an educational context is to make a judgement about mastery of skills or knowledge; to measure improvement over time; to arrive at some definitions of strengths and weaknesses; to rank people for selection or exclusion, or perhaps to motivate them.'

(Postgraduate Medical Education and Training Board)

Evaluation: 'Evaluation is the collection of, analysis and interpretation of information about any aspect of a programme of education or training as part of a recognised process of judging its effectiveness, its efficiency and any other outcomes it may have.'
(Thorpe 1993)

Both curricula and competencies may be articulated into specific **learning outcomes** (what is expected to be learned) and/or **learning objectives** (what and how learning takes place) (see Chapter 2). A short course, for example, is likely to have an overall aim to improve competence or educate in a particular area and some specific objectives that indicate what learning should take place.

Consider a two-hour first aid course. The overall aim will be to help the learner to be better at, or more informed about, delivering first aid. Within this there may be specific learning outcomes such as:

1 Be able to identify the appropriateness of cardiopulmonary resuscitation (CPR) for a person who is unconscious
2 Be able to deliver CPR when appropriate.

In general, assessment should relate to specific indicators of what learning or level of competence is expected. In the absence of these, learning outcomes can be derived from the overall aims or curriculum of the learning programme.

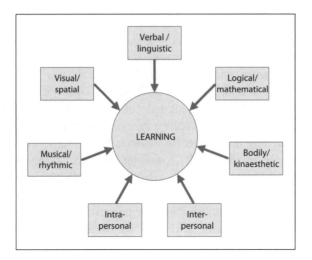

Figure 4.2. Multiple intelligences. (Adapted from Gardner 1983.)

In some instances the aims, learning outcomes and learning objectives may be defined by the learner (consider again the PhD thesis and viva). However, if the learning aims or objectives are not defined when they are expected to be, are defined poorly, or do not relate well to the work undertaken, this will very likely be a criticism by examiners.

The examples of assessment detailed in this chapter focus on cognitive ability, but it is worth remembering other aspects of performance that may be assessed, such as physical ability or interpersonal skills (see Fig. 4.2). Taking again the example of the first aid course, assessment could demonstrate cognitive recall of information as well as competence in enacting a typical first aid scenario. However, concepts that are demonstrated physically may also be assessed theoretically – a chemical titration that exhibits a colour change can be described regardless of whether it is actually conducted. Indeed, assessment may be used to quantify or qualify learning that is difficult to demonstrate but can be described instead.

How assessment meets learning

In an ideal world the best assessment would be one that most fairly reflects the learning, competence or performance of an individual. However, apart from the practical constraints of time and personnel, we must also appreciate that no method of assessment will assess the entirety of what has been, or is being, learned. People exhibit different characteristics and intelligences – be they learned or innate – and develop different **learning styles** and strategies. (See Chapter 2 for more information on learning styles.)

Some people may rely on memory and recall whereas others may rely on conceptual thinking or 'stories'. Any given assessment will have a bias in some way towards a particular learning style or even human characteristic. Therefore, rather than trying to suit the 'horse to the course' (which could be criticised as being unfair in itself and impossible anyway) it is worth at least trying to create a level playing field in delivering assessments.

One way of doing this is to create a mix of different assessment methods that measure learning from different aspects. This can also give the assessor greater confidence in the results, provided that the assessment methods are robust and are truly measuring what is intended. Sometimes only one assessment method will be suitable to measure a very specific element of learning. Similarly, there will be some aspects of learning that cannot be assessed accurately or reliably. Although we should strive to be creative in our methods, this has to be an accepted limitation.

The assessor

The role of the assessor is very important. There ought to be objectivity in relation to the learner, whether they come face-to-face or not. There should be no conflict of interest, in order to eliminate positive or negative bias. This can be tricky as in some circumstances the ideal person to assess is the person who is closest to the learner's practice or performance. As an assessor you should ask yourself, do you have multiple interests in the outcome of the assessment that may impact on its outcome? Discussion with colleagues or the human resources team could help to answer this.

The roles and responsibilities of the assessor are varied. Again, in the absence of guidelines or a pre-defined set of answers, it is helpful to consider the purpose of the assessment and focus on the learning objectives to clarify what should be assessed. If the assessor plays an active part in the interpretation of the learner's responses then some degree of competence on the assessor's part and/or familiarity with both the assessment method and responses may be expected. Indeed, specialist assessors may be specifically recruited to perform or mark the assessment.

Assessment value

How do you know whether your judgement of a learner's performance is accurate? Of course there is often subjectivity in assessment and assessors must ensure that outcomes can be reproduced to a standard degree of error (that is, different assessors will give similar marks). Even if the assessment is a **subjective assessment** there may be some structured criteria and recording format that you are expected to follow in order to provide feedback, either for the learner or for quality assurance purposes. If the outcome of the assessment is a quantitative mark or percentage, the question arises of what

Table 4.1 Objective and subjective rating scores							
Criterion	Highly competent		Competent		Not yet competent/ does not meet minimum criteria		Unacceptable
Overall ability	Evidence presented *substantially* exceeds minimum requirements of competence in terms of content, structure, knowledge, insight and other defined criteria		Evidence presented is a sufficient, valid, reliable indication that the learner has met minimum requirements of competence		Evidence presented indicates that the learner has not yet demonstrated overall competence or is not yet competent in terms of one or more of the specified criteria		Evidence presented is substantially flawed, gross inaccuracies, omissions, irrelevant content or substantial deviation from the specified criteria
	Excellent	Very good	Good; Com-petent	Satisfactory	Just below standard	Weak	Very weak	Very little of relevance
Mark earned	85–100%	75%	65%	55%	45%	35%	25%	0–15%

this actually means or equates to. This may be easier to judge if there is a pass mark or if percentage points are categorised into different levels of proficiency.

An example of objective and subjective scoring is shown in Table 4.1. There is subjective categorisation and there are equivalent descriptions of levels of competence and percentage scores.

It is also worth remembering that the value of the outcome may only be valid for a period of time. The significance of any achievement is likely to decrease over time or through greater achievements. For example, it is likely that qualifications achieved at school are superseded by university qualifications, and they in turn by professional qualifications – although basic, lower-level qualifications may still be required to demonstrate proficiency in core subjects such as English and mathematics. If there is a specific expiry date, it may relate to ensuring that individuals are up-to-date in their learning or competence – consider again the first aid course.

So how can we ensure that assessments are a true reflection of performance? In the United Kingdom there is annual debate following the release of key school examination results concerning their validity. As results continue to improve year on year, the media perception is that the examinations are getting easier. In certain circumstances, particularly where one is being measured against one's own previous performance in formative assessments, this is irrelevant – you would expect and hope to see improvement over time.

However, there may be justification for reviewing a cohort of results by analysing, for example, the 'average' score (mean/median/mode), the standard deviation from the mean, and any outlying results that may have a disproportionate effect on the average. How does this year's analysis compare with those of the previous year(s)? Are there any patterns? If so, can these patterns be explained? How will this inform how we assess next year?

If the assessment method included a battery of questions or 'items', such as the MCQ, a technique called a **'test-item analysis'** may be employed, particularly in an academic setting. This judges each item against pre-defined external criteria or against the remaining items in the assessment. In performing this analysis, there may be one item that is consistently answered incorrectly or not answered at all, even by the highest scorers. This raises suspicion as to whether the question was fair or whether it could be reasonably interpreted in a number of ways.

Two outcomes may result from the analysis. One is the *post-hoc* improvement in the assessment questions or items. The second is adjustment to the assessment scores to reflect the difficulty or fairness of the assessment. If the second option is used, it should be done consistently (i.e. with every assessment of its kind) and in a disciplined way against agreed criteria in order to avoid accusations of manipulating results.

Feedback on assessment

The question of how the outcome of assessment is fed back to the learner again relates to the nature of the assessment. If the assessment is formative, it is likely that learners will receive feedback in order to guide future learning (see Fig. 4.3). However, if the outcome of the assessment is summative, feedback may not be given – often not even under appeal – especially if the desired outcome is achieved. This usually relates to the practical balance of providing feedback versus the transparency of the academic process. Academics need to be transparent, but the reality of providing hundreds or thousands of individuals with detailed feedback is not viable. However, educational institutions will typically have processes in place for appeal and re-marking even if feedback is not granted.

There is also the danger of conflict if assessment is heavily subjective and the learner disagrees with the assessor's interpretation; this is not easily managed on a large scale.

Setting

The setting or venue for an assessment is also important. The setting may not be decided until the day of the actual assessment, for example if it is a work-based observation. In this instance the assessor should always take

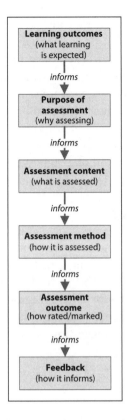

Figure 4.3. The process of assessment.

the lead in ensuring that the setting is appropriate. Is there enough space? Is it too busy or noisy to properly conduct an assessment? If patients or members of the public are involved, are there any confidentiality issues? Is it possible to provide feedback within this setting if it is required?

Plagiarism in assessment

It is extremely important to recognise the significance of plagiarism in assessment as the risk of accrediting learning that has not taken place could result in tangible damage even to human life. Individual institutions will provide their own guidance relating to plagiarism in assessment and we refer the reader to these institutional policies and practices. The process for tackling plagiarism should nonetheless be consistent, fair and transparent. However, the message to be encouraged regarding plagiarism is that it is never in the learner's interests, regardless of whether it is detected or not. In particular, with formative assessment – where the only direct benefit is to the learner – plagiarism defeats the purpose of this method and therefore actually disadvantages the learner.

It should also be recognised that plagiarism is not always intentional. For example, learners may not be aware that they must reference texts or quotations that they have used. There is a need for clear understanding at the commencement of learning as to what plagiarism encompasses. At this stage it is also advisable to encourage an open culture of reporting plagiarism to ease detection. There are a number of detection methods and any one method should not be relied upon. With the increasingly broad range of assessment methodologies there is a need for detection methods to respond. For further information on plagiarism see the good practice guide by Carroll and Appleton (2001).

Methods of assessment

A vast battery of assessment methods have emerged that seek to provide a means of quantifying and articulating learning. The following methods have been selected to demonstrate the broad field of tools that can be applied in different learning settings and for different reasons; for example, some that are competency-based and some that are not. The list does not seek to be exhaustive – further reading suggestions can be found at the end of the chapter.

Essay

Essays are a common method of formal assessment, especially in the academic field. Written from the perspective of the author, they usually offer critique or argument around a central theme. Examples of types of essay include short-answer essays, standard essays, extended-time essays, and dissertations (see Miller *et al.* 1998). For the purposes of assessment this theme may be posed as a question or statement to which the learner responds. When setting an essay as an assessment you may like to consider the following:

- Is an essay the most appropriate form of assessment to use? Consider the skills and resources that are required for essay writing and assessment.
- How important is it that the essay is written in an invigilated setting? Consider the risk of plagiarism and the extent to which sources or evidence need to be referred to.
- Is the essay being used as a summative or formative assessment? This may inform the degree of feedback that is required or desired.

There is a great degree of flexibility and subjectivity that can be daunting both for the learner and the assessor. However, in broad terms, there are a number of criteria against which an essay can be judged. When marking an essay, consider the following points:

- Does the title bear relation to the text?
- Is the essay well constructed and organised? Consider the use of paragraphs.
- Is the argument or perspective obvious?
- Is there a clear beginning and end?
- Is there balance – has the opposing view or breadth of evidence been considered and debated?
- Is there reference to source materials/evidence? Has this evidence been accurately or appropriately presented in the context of the essay? Has it been critically appraised?
- Is there a consistent approach to detail?
- If there were time constraints, has this impacted on the content or flow of the essay?

When deciding on a grade for an essay, think about the following (see also Table 4.2):

- Skim-read the essay, making brief notes to follow up with a more thorough reading and analysis of the essay.
- Provide constructive feedback or critique. For example, write a summary of the essay. This 'back-translation' will show the writer how the essay was understood (or not). List key stronger and weaker points and explain your reasoning. Play the 'devil's advocate', especially if the opposing view is lacking.
- Allow yourself to give the essay the time and attention it needs to provide a fair assessment. Consider any conflicts of interest you might have (for example, an opposing view to your own!).
- Refer to relevant local guidelines.

Multiple Choice Question (MCQ) assessment

For facts that can be efficiently administered and marked, and whose validity can be objectively evaluated, the **MCQ** remains a popular and common form of assessment. However, there are a number of limitations to the various forms of MCQ assessment and it is worth considering these. The two main forms of MCQ are the True/False format and the 'single-best answer' family. Although other formats exist, all are characterised by a question or statement and a series of possible answers to which the learner responds.

True/False format: The learner indicates whether the possible answers to a question or statement are true or false (Box 4.2). Limitations of this format include guessing and cueing (using the process of elimination). Negative marking (removing points for wrong answers) can be used to suppress guessing, but this in turn has an impact. Females may generally have a

Table 4.2 Essay assessment criteria

Degree grade	Per cent score	Descriptor
'First' (I)	>70	Thorough understanding of key concepts/theory. Relevant and effective use of material. Evidence of wide reading with critical understanding. Relevant synthesis of material. Independence of thought and argument. Well-structured, fluent argument. Clear, correct and accomplished writing.
2-1 (II-i)	60–69	A good, if imperfect, grasp of the material and its implications. Identifies the focus of the question. Knowledge and clear understanding of contrasting viewpoints. Generally clear and correct writing. A case well argued and convincingly presented.
2-2 (II-ii)	50–59	A reasonable grasp of the material. A general ability to present relevant argument but might contain some irrelevant material. Some coherent argument but weaknesses in overall structure and clarity.
'Third' (III)	40–49	A basic grasp of the material, marred by either poor discriminative ability, an element of conceptual naivety, or both. Tendency to unsubstantiated statements/assertions. Shallow interpretation. May contain significant errors of fact or interpretation. Some understanding of class material, but little or no further reading. Little evidence of independent thought. Poorly structured and presented, with little coherent argument.
Fail	<40	Does not satisfy the minimum requirements for the exercise in question. Little understanding, even of class material. No structure. Does not address the topic.

[a] Based on guidelines from University of Hertfordshire (see Resources).

negative bias as they are less likely to risk guessing. This form of assessment has largely been abandoned in the United States but is still common in the United Kingdom.

Single Best Answer format: The learner selects the correct answer from a number of possible answers (Box 4.3). With this format the cueing effect is reduced with the use of a greater number of possible answers in extended-matching questions (EMQs). EMQs increase the reliability and discriminatory power of this format.

Viva

A **viva** (viva voce examination) is, by definition, an oral assessment. Similarly to an interview, the learner will usually face a panel of examiners who will question and discuss with the learner the work that is being examined. The purpose of the viva is usually either as part of a structured assessment schedule, for example against written work (a thesis or dissertation), or as an exception to normal circumstances, for example to correctly categorise borderline cases.

> *Box 4.2* *Example of True/False format MCQ*
>
> *Which of the following statements about tuberculosis (TB) are CORRECT?:*
>
> **1** TB is caused by a virus. [False]
> **2** TB only infects the lungs. [False]
> **3** A range of diagnostic techniques including chest X-ray, sputum smear microscopy and sputum smear culture are used in diagnosis of TB. [True]
> **4** TB is more common in individuals who have suppressed immune systems. [True]
> **5** If an individual has been cured of TB it is impossible for them to contract the disease again. [False]

There will usually be guidelines or regulations for the procedure of conducting a viva, including the preparation of materials beforehand and how to communicate the outcome of the viva to the student. It is important to be familiar with the system used at any particular institution.

Common assessment methods used in health professions education

Fig. 4.1 at the beginning of the chapter showed some commonly used generic methods of assessment. However, there are some specific methods used to assess healthcare students that can particularly focus on clinical competence (see Fig. 4.4 for an overview).

Mini Clinical Evaluation Exercise (mini-CEX)

Originally created by the American Board of Internal Medicine, the Mini Clinical Evaluation Exercise (**mini-CEX**) assesses a practitioner 'one-to-one' in the context of their clinical environment. The focus of this method is on the observation of the clinical skills, attitudes and behaviours of the learner in practitioner–patient interactions.

The mini-CEX has been adapted for different contexts and therefore may assess against specific objectives or learning outcomes. However, general themes that will always be assessed include:

- Ability to communicate effectively
- Appropriate use of information
- Professional/clinical judgement
- Appropriate outcome reached.

> **Box 4.3** *Example of Single Best Answer format MCQ*
>
> A 72-year-old woman visits her family doctor complaining of pain in her arm when she walks the dog. Investigations show that she has a high cholesterol level and hypertension, and is an ex-smoker (50 cigarettes a day for 40 years). She is diagnosed with stable angina. Which of the following medicines is inappropriate in her treatment for stable angina?
>
> **1** Sublingual glyceryl trinitrate
> **2** Atenolol
> **3** Aspirin
> **4** Digoxin

Key features of the mini-CEX

- It is observed and assessed by an experienced practitioner.
- It involves real-life encounter, for example on a hospital ward or outpatient clinic.
- It uses prospective assessment in real time; 'thinking on your feet' problem solving.
- It is designed specifically for clinical emphasis.
- The assessor does not need to know the learner.
- Structured feedback – vocal and written – is given; used as reference and evidence of progression
- The duration is typically 15–20 min (including time for feedback).
- The frequency depends on the learning programme but over a six-month period a minimum of three occasions would be feasible and provide a 'direction of travel' in terms of measuring learning progression.
- It can use a range of assessors in different contexts.

Case-Based Discussion (CBD)

The **Case-Based Discussion** (CBD) was developed to assess clinical judgement, decision-making and application of knowledge. As with the mini-CEX, the CBD is context-specific and has been adapted for various uses in clinical settings. However, universally it provides the opportunity to explore and probe the learner's deeper understanding and knowledge of specific issues from a professional perspective. This involves a structured 'one-to-one' in-depth discussion, between an experienced practitioner (the assessor) and the learner, of a clinical event with which the learner was intrinsically involved.

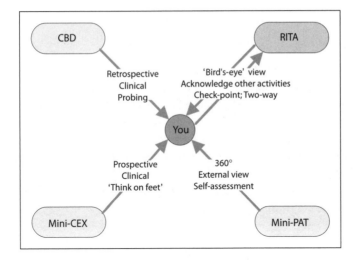

Figure 4.4. Methods of assessment often used with healthcare students.

Key features of the CBD

- It is assessed by an experienced practitioner.
- It involves real-life encounter, for example clinical cases from a hospital ward or outpatient clinic.
- It uses retrospective assessment: recall of information, documentation, reflection on decision/actions.
- It is designed specifically for clinical emphasis.
- The assessor does not need to know the learner.
- Structured discussion and feedback – vocal and written – are given; used as reference and evidence of progression.
- The duration is typically 15–20 min (including time for feedback).
- The frequency of assessment depends on learning programme, but over a six-month period a minimum of three occasions would be feasible and would provide a 'direction of travel' in terms of measuring learning progression.
- It uses a range of assessors in different contexts.

Mini Peer Assessment Tool (Mini-PAT)

Developed from the Sheffield Peer Review Tool (SPRAT), the Mini Peer Assessment Tool (**mini-PAT**) is sometimes referred to as a **360 degree assessment,** in that it should reflect feedback on a learner both from their own perspective and from the spectrum of co-workers who witness the learner's performance and practice. These co-workers are nominated by the learner to provide anonymous feedback on their performance over a period of time.

Personal view 4.1 The mini-CEX

Background/preparation

Jon was a junior pharmacist who had recently started a new six-month clinical rotation on a hospital ward (care of the elderly). As part of the allied diploma he was enrolled in he had to complete three mini-CEX assessments in his current rotation.

Jon and I agreed on a suitable time and date for an assessment on the ward – there was typically a dip in the workload on Wednesdays when Jon usually worked on his continuing professional development (CPD).

The mini-CEX

On Wednesday I joined Jon on the ward after he had selected three new patients. I had a quick look through the medical notes and selected one of the cases. We went to the patient's bedside, where Jon asked the patient's permission if I observed him while he took his medication history. The patient agreed and Jon began his consultation. I positioned myself discreetly and made some notes on the mini-CEX forms provided (Jon's details, the setting, the patient's details) and focused on Jon's ability to take an accurate medication history from the patient. At the end of the consultation, we both thanked the patient.

Feedback and reflection

I began by asking Jon what he believed went well and then questioned him about his clinical encounter. In particular, we discussed an unusual medicine that was prescribed and I asked Jon to reflect on whether he chose the most appropriate action and what other options he considered.

We agreed strengths and areas for improvement along with an action plan to capitalise on Jon's learning. We summarised our discussions and actions in the necessary paperwork and Jon added this to his Portfolio of Evidence folder.

The next time Jon completes a mini-CEX he will be able to compare his progress and this will form part of the discussions.

Sue, education and training manager

The nominees then rate the learner under a set of criteria – delivery of patient care, personal attributes, and so on. This assessment works best if managed electronically to collect feedback. Results are collated to show the learner's self-evaluation against mean responses of their co-workers and against a

Personal view 4.2 The CBD

Background/preparation

Shahida was a junior medical resident coming to the end of a four-month surgical placement. As part of the hospital work-based assessment programme she had to complete two CBDs. However, as the two she had already completed were in very different settings, she wanted to complete a third before the end of her placement to better demonstrate her progress.

The CBD

We agreed that she would complete a CBD one afternoon and she presented me with three possible cases for discussion. I chose a critical incident that Shahida had been involved in and began by asking her to give a summary of the case, including any relevant documentation, and what motivated her actions. During the discussion I probed Shahida's knowledge around diagnoses of the case involved and the implications of the delayed diagnosis that resulted in the critical incident. I finished the discussion by referring directly to Shahida's learning syllabus as a standard in gauging her progression throughout the placement.

Feedback and reflection

We both agreed on, and documented on the accompanying CBD forms, areas that Shahida needed to focus on before she left her placement, as well as more generally as she progresses. However, I was also keen to emphasise the progress that Shahida had made in comparison with her previous CBDs and how this could be taken forward in terms of her career decisions. This formed the basis for the action plan we formed.

Paul, consultant trainer

mean score for a cohort of learners that they belong to (for example, other students). A tutor or supervisor feeds back the results and discusses them with the learner, agreeing strengths and key areas for improvement.

Key features of the mini-PAT

- It is assessed by a range of co-workers.
- There is aggregation of feedback to compare co-workers' scores with self-scoring and student group scores.
- The assessors need to be familiar with the performance or practice of the learner.

- Discussion and feedback with a tutor are given with reference to score analysis.
- Completing the mini-PAT typically takes 15–20 min; feedback typically takes 15–20 min.
- The frequency of assessment depends on learning programme but can be once per module or course; best done around the midpoint to guide learning.
- It uses of a range of assessors in different contexts.

Record of In-Training Assessment (RITA)

The **Record of In-Training Assessment** (RITA) was intended as an annual 'stop-check' on progress to ensure standards of training by assessing against a set of criteria. This is supported by a portfolio of evidence detailing an individual's activities and learning. An interview between the learner and their supervisor is performed. The outcome is essentially to identify whether there is any cause for concern regarding the individual and also to articulate a plan of action for future progress. The RITA has been adapted for use in different areas and can bring together the various ongoing assessments as part of the evidence presented in a portfolio to evaluate progress.

Key features of the RITA

- It is a 'stop-check' to review progress, not an assessment in itself, but it brings together the learner's evidence of progress including formative ongoing assessments.
- It is retrospective; it relies on a portfolio of evidence presented by the learner and discussion during the interview.
- It is assessed by an experienced practitioner familiar with the learner.
- Structured discussion and feedback – vocal and written – are given; feedback is used to direct the learner, for example, using targets or goals.
- No mark or grade is given, but it documents progress and achievements.
- The duration is typically 45 min (including time for feedback).
- The frequency: depends on 'course' or rotation duration. Typically conduct one RITA at the midpoint of each rotation.

Objective Structured Clinical Examination (OSCE)

The **Objective Structured Clinical Examination** (OSCE) aims to assess not only knowledge and attitudes but also communication and practical skills. Oriented around a station-based system, the focus of assessment changes with each station. For example, a medical OSCE may focus separately

Personal view 4.3   *The mini-PAT*

Background/preparation

Sunni was a physiotherapist working in the community setting studying towards a postgraduate certificate course. As part of her studies she was required to gain feedback midway through by completing the mini-PAT.

Sunni selected and contacted a number of her colleagues who had observed her practice. She nominated them electronically to give feedback on her practice.

The mini-PAT

Sunni had selected four of her physiotherapy colleagues including her line manager to complete the mini-PAT. She had also selected a physician and two practice nurses, as well as the physiotherapy assistant with whom she worked closely.

All the nominees received email invitations to complete the mini-PAT assessment for Sunni. Sunni also received the mini-PAT to complete a self-evaluation.

Feedback and reflection

As Sunni's practice tutor I received the results of Sunni's mini-PAT assessment and arranged to review them with her. I began by asking Sunni what she thought the feedback would look like and how she perceived her strengths and areas of improvement. We then looked at the results. Sunni seemed quite nervous. We focused especially on areas where Sunni's self-rating deviated from either what her co-workers had fed back or from her certificate group mean score. Sunni consistently rated herself below the ratings of her co-workers, who generally scored her higher than the certificate group mean. There were some areas for improvement, especially around communication, but overall the feedback was very positive.

I suggested to Sunni that she might be lacking in self-confidence and she agreed that this did hinder her communication. We planned a strategy to give her more exposure to colleagues and I suggested that Sunni look for opportunities to 'shadow' her senior colleagues in leadership positions.

Maria, practice tutor

on patient history of disease, examination, investigations and treatment. The learner moves in sequence through the timed stations, which may be

Personal view 4.4 The RITA

Background/preparation

Siegfried is a junior nurse who has enrolled on a six-month infectious diseases course offered by the local university. This requires an evaluation of progress halfway through, using the RITA. Siegfried has had some concerns with fitting the work associated with this academic course into his day-to-day work as a nurse. He is looking forward to the RITA as a chance to discuss his progress and concerns. He compiles his portfolio of evidence and realises that it is quite sparse – he has attended all the course lectures but has only completed a few case studies of relevant patients in addition to this. He arranges to meet his course tutor after one of the lectures.

The RITA

The interview starts well as Siegfried is an enthusiastic student. However, when I turn to his portfolio, I am disappointed and would have expected to see more. Siegfried agrees but says he finds it difficult to gather formal evidence in his job. Together we plan how Siegfried will meet the expectations of learning for the course and how he will demonstrate this. I remind Siegfried of the formative assessments and that he should arrange with his practice supervisor in his workplace to complete these.

Feedback and reflection

We fill in a RITA form together after agreeing a course of action. This will inform the practice supervisor of my concerns. Siegfried plans to complete one assessment a week as well as writing up some more case studies. He will then communicate his actions to both me as, his academic tutor, and his workplace supervisor in about a month's time.

Siobhan, academic tutor

manned or unmanned. Props may be used to re-create or simulate real-life experiences. For example, this may require interaction with actors playing the roles of healthcare professionals or patients. However, by having the learner sit a number of different stations, under time constraints, it is intended to provide a broad appraisal of the knowledge, skills and attitudes desired. This will involve more than the provision of the correct answer such as identifying a treatment issue. Hence, you can expect that all manned OSCE stations will require a basic level of communication including, for

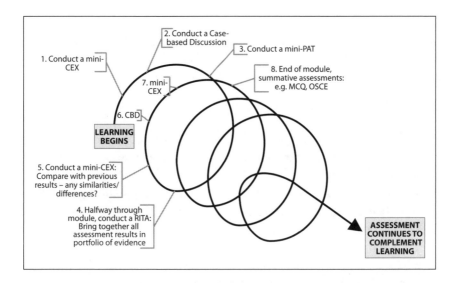

Figure 4.5. An example of assessment of learning through ongoing formative and summative methods.

example, a clear introduction by the learner and a degree of professionalism. Look in Appendix 4 for an example of an OSCE.

Competency frameworks

Assessments may be directly linked with competency frameworks. For example, an assessment that is used in postgraduate pharmacy education in England called the 'General Level Framework' (GLF) was developed to articulate the National Health Service Knowledge and Skills Framework (NHS KSF), which was intended to provide an objective framework to identify knowledge and skills, and to develop public healthcare workers.

Closing the loop

Learning can be seen as a cyclical process through formal structured education or training courses and degrees, as well as life experiences (see Fig. 4.5). Given a start and an end point, in a structured learning process the learning can be assessed using the tools described above, which seek to complement each other in what they assess as well as their purpose of assessment. The aim of assessment, therefore, should be one of supporting learning as well as a process or method of judging the progress or outcome of learning.

Summary

This chapter has introduced you to a variety of assessment methods for use in both the academic and healthcare practice fields. Some you may be familiar with and some may be new to you. More than one method can be used in concert to deliver robust assessment that is fair, reliable and pragmatic. Assessment should be considered throughout the learning experience, not just as an end point but as an aid to learning.

Top tips

- Research and understand the assessment methods to be able to defend or critique your choice or the choice placed upon you.
- Choose the fairest method of assessment that is practical.
- Consider what is achievable, not just the least amount of work.
- Relate assessment methods to the objectives or competencies of the curriculum or workplace.
- Explain to your learners the purpose of any given assessment.
- Try to use a combination of assessment methods that best complement each other wherever possible.
- Encourage a culture of learning through assessment rather than assessment as an ominous end point.

Exercise 4.1 What is the primary reason for the assessment you are involved in?

- Informing future learning
- Indicating past learning
- As a management tool
- To identify incompetence or reward competence
- As a selection method
- As a motivational tool
- Other

References and further reading

Archer J *et al.* (2008). Mini-PAT (Peer Assessment Tool): a valid component of a national assessment programme in the UK? *Advances in Health Sciences Education: Theory and Practice* **13**(2): 181–192.

Carroll J, Appleton J (2001). *Plagiarism. A Good Practice Guide.* Oxford: Joint Information Systems Committee. Oxford Brookes University.

Feather A *et al.* (2004). *OSCEs for Medical Students: Volume 1.* Knutsford: PasTest.

Gardner H (1983). *Frames of Mind: The Theory of Multiple Intelligences.* New York: Basic Books.

Gibbs G (1995). *Improving Student Learning through Assessment and Evaluation.* Oxford: Oxford Centre for Staff Development.

Irons A (2008). *Enhancing Learning through Formative Assessment and Feedback.* Oxford: Routledge.

Joint Programmes Board (2009). *Assessment Handbook*. London. www.jpbsoutheast.org/about/.

Miller AH *et al.* (1998). *Student Assessment in Higher Education: A Handbook for Assessing Performance*. London: Kogan Page.

Nathenson MB, Henderson ES (1980). *Using Student Feedback to Improve Learning Materials*. Woking: Biddles.

Rowntree D (1987). *Assessing Students: How Shall We Know Them?* London: Kogan Page.

Thorpe M (1993). In: Ellington H *et al.*, eds. *Handbook of Educational Technology*. London: Kogan Page.

Resources

National Board of Medical Examiners (Philadelphia). www.nbme.org/index.html.

Assessment Policies & Procedures (Robert Gordon University, UK). www.rgu.ac.uk/academicaffairs/assessment.

Essay assessment criteria (University of Hertfordshire, UK). www.herts.ac.uk/courses/schools-of-study/humanities/subject-areas/philosophy/subject-guide/essay-assessment-criteria.cfm.

Intercollegiate Surgical Curriculum Programme. Assessment and Feedback. *Overview of the Assessment System*. www.iscp.ac.uk/Assessment.

5

Evaluating teaching

Tina Brock

So far in this text, you have learned about developing a teaching philosophy, planning for teaching activities, developing instructional materials, and assessing learning. But how will you know whether all this hard work has yielded the results you are expecting? This chapter discusses how to evaluate your effectiveness as a teacher and improve your teaching based on this information. This is a critical part of professional development for both the full-time educator and the health professional with educational responsibilities. The chapter begins with a discussion of some of the methods available for teachers to evaluate their performance in teaching sessions. It then focuses on using the information collected to re-design a course or activity. It concludes with a summary of the major concepts including top tips to guide you.

How will you know if you are achieving your teaching goals?

Most individuals attracted to careers as teachers, in particular those in the healthcare arena, are quality conscious and want to do the very best job possible. But while we become comfortable assessing the work of our students and the scientific community at large, it is not always natural (or pleasant) to put our own performance under the same microscope.

It is important to realise that, despite the best intentions and careful preparation, it is reasonable to expect that not every teaching technique, course activity and assessment procedure will be 100% successful, particularly the first time we try it. This may be the result of a variety of factors ... and even just bad luck (see Box 5.1). But if we are to remain in harmony with the teaching philosophy we have developed as well as continuously improve our teaching (reaping the benefits of all the hard work invested in the concepts discussed in Chapters 1 to 4 of this text), it is important to establish a systematic way to know which teaching methods are most powerful (leading to sustained improvements in knowledge, skills and attitudes), and most efficient (making the best use of your time).

> *Box 5.1* *Categories of common barriers to teaching effectiveness*
>
> - *Systemic* – for example, teaching is not a valued activity within the organisation
> - *External* – for example, the learners have not mastered concepts foundational to the current discussion
> - *Internal* – for example, the teacher speaks in a very quiet voice in a large lecture hall
> - *Serendipitous* – for example, the activity is scheduled late in the afternoon just prior to a school holiday

This is similar to the experience of a clinician monitoring the effectiveness of a combination treatment for diabetes (for example, diet, exercise and medications). After one month of care, does the patient's health status improve? If so, what is the reason for this? Would you advise that the therapy be continued in the same way or changed to a different treatment?

To answer these questions, the clinician would likely interview the patient, order and review the results of specific laboratory tests, compare the situation with evidence found in the literature, and perhaps talk to a few colleagues about the case. Likewise, teachers in the healthcare professions must be able to 'diagnose' challenges using a variety of specific tools. Following this, they can target and monitor educational 'treatments' based on this information.

Who should drive the evaluation process?

Looking at educational systems holistically, the degree of organisational support (i.e. that provided by deans, department chairs, and other programmatic leaders) is a good predictor for teaching quality. Ideally, some form of summative teaching evaluation will be required by an employer as part of annual review or for consideration of promotion or merit award. If this is so, there may be predetermined processes (e.g. end-of-course surveys; see Appendix 7) in which all teachers participate. These can be very helpful but if not planned carefully, supported, and used consistently by the leadership of the organisation, they may not be taken seriously. Indeed, over time, review systems can become somewhat 'mechanised'; that is, the process is completed only because it is required, not because it is valued as a way to improve teaching.

Even in the best systems, however, to truly be prepared to make timely changes in a course, some teacher-initiated formative evaluation will also likely be necessary (see Chapter 4 for more explanation of summative and formative review and Appendices 5 to 8 for sample instruments). This means that the person who should drive the evaluation process is also the person who has the most to gain from it – you!

What are the types and sources of information for evaluation?

Just as in conducting a scientific experiment, there are two types of data that can be used to evaluate the effectiveness of a teaching session – namely, opinions and facts. Both types are important for comprehensive evaluation but each gives you a different type of information useful in becoming the most effective teacher possible. In addition, there are multiple sources from which you can collect these opinions and facts.

Opinions

Opinions about the teaching session may be generated via self-reflection, from the learners, and from peers in the teaching process.

Reflection

Reflection will be discussed in more detail in Chapter 6, but for now you should know that one of the most efficient ways to monitor your teaching involves making systematic notes about your experiences. These can be done manually, just jotting down notes in a diary, or electronically using a variety of computer programs. Some teachers recommend starting with your initial feelings or impressions then reviewing these periodically to develop more structured summaries (see Appendices 5 to 8).

For this to be most effective, it is important to make time for this activity immediately after each teaching session. You may think you will be able to remember all the important details of your teaching (how much additional time was needed to clarify a particular concept, for example), but as the teaching sessions add up over the term, the ability to recall these issues in detail (even the traumatic ones) diminishes.

When reflecting, it is important to include your thoughts about both what went well, and what could be improved. See Appendix 3 for one example of how to include this in a regular lesson plan and Chapter 6 for more specifics about how to get started with reflection.

If you reflect consistently, over time you will likely notice a pattern to the types of activities that are documented as most compatible with your innate teaching style. And when you bring more of this to your teaching, you will naturally feel more comfortable in the role.

Learners

Another source of opinion is that of the learner. This may take the form of teacher evaluations (such as perceptions about the teacher's readiness and availability) or course evaluations (such as perceptions of the effectiveness

> *Box 5.2   Is learner feedback just a popularity contest?*
>
> Not if managed appropriately!
>
> There is some evidence to suggest that learners pay more attention to and engage more with concepts, methods or materials that they 'like', and for this reason it is beneficial to know what they like.
>
> But there are concepts that are critical and foundational, regardless of whether they are particularly well-liked by the learners. For these important concepts, you should look for other strategies with which to engage the learner.

of the course or practical clinical experience). These are usually the most common form of teaching evaluation.

Some critics have called learner ratings both 'overemphasised' and 'underutilised', so before proceeding it is important to note that learner feedback is very important but it should never be considered the sole source of information or in raw format. Rather, it should be included as one part of a comprehensive evaluation (some evidence suggests that learner ratings should contribute 30–50% of the total teaching evaluation), and should include both an introduction to describe the methods and explanation to interpret the results. Neglecting to include this explanatory information along with learner evaluation data would be like a clinician trying to evaluate a clinical laboratory result without knowing the laboratory's reference range for that test – the information is just not meaningful.

When collecting feedback from learners it is usually more helpful to focus their attention on *process* rather than *content*. For example, a learner in the preliminary years of a particular course may lack the professional insight to be able to consider the future usefulness of a specific content area. This can manifest as comments such as 'I'll never need to know about X, so it should be removed from the curriculum', particularly when the topic in question is especially challenging or is competing with a more popular or more clearly mapped topic (see Box 5.2).

Because the *content* areas for most courses are (or should be) linked directly to curricular outcomes for the entire programme (also known as the curricular map), individual teachers may have less influence (at the course level) on the inclusion of specific topic areas. This suggests that spending precious evaluation time collecting learner feedback about content areas may just be frustrating for all involved.

In general, learners are *not* well equipped to judge things such as:

- The appropriateness of the content and objectives

- The teacher's knowledge of the subject matter
- The degree to which the material reflects current information
- The appropriateness of the grading standards.

But learners *are* especially valuable in providing feedback regarding the instructional process itself, including:

- The amount of time spent on a particular concept relative to its importance in the course objectives
- The types of exercises used to promote mastery of a concept
- Characteristics of the classroom dynamic or learning environment.

In fact, learner input on these latter aspects is critical as they can offer the perspective of someone naive to the content area, as opposed to that of an expert. It is true that often once a subject is mastered (as by a teacher), it can be difficult to remember what it was like 'not to know' and, in these cases, learner input can ensure that discussions are directed at or build from the appropriate level.

The *process* for collecting feedback from learners may be formal or informal. As mentioned earlier, many programmes will have some sort of formal, summative review process allowing learners to provide feedback anonymously at the end of all courses. This may take the form of standardised surveys or item banks from which teachers can select questions in order to build semi-customised surveys. It may even include support for analysis of the responses such as the ability to compare results across disciplines or ranks.

The literature describes the pros and cons of such systems, with particular attention paid to the lack of validity and reliability of many of these locally-developed ratings tools. This scientific challenge can cause faculty support for such systems to be quite low and perhaps compromise your ability to use the results to promote change. Still, if your university or health facility requires this type of end-of-teaching evaluation, it will be difficult not to comply regardless of the limitations and you should do your best to optimise whatever programmatic resources are available.

Recognising the potential flaws of the instruments described above as well as the constraints of the systems (e.g. time lag), to be most useful the summative evaluation process should be augmented with more formative methods (see Appendices 5 to 8). In fact, using a mid-term evaluation to collect rapid feedback from learners can provide the teacher with time to address any critical issues quickly, as well as to develop a plan for more extensive changes before the next course offering. In addition, teachers who routinely collect and use interim learner evaluation information are typically rated as more learner-centred.

If you are planning to collect your own learner feedback, what mechanism should you use? Techniques such as 'minute papers', in which, for example, at the conclusion of a specific lecture the teacher asks the learners

> *Box 5.3   Resist the temptation!*
>
> The internet includes a growing number of sites that allow spontaneous 'rating' of teachers (e.g. RateMyProfessors.com). While we respect the learner's freedom to 'vent' frustrations, many of the comments on these sites are not designed to be constructive and some are inappropriate. Since you cannot un-know this kind of 'feedback', this is one distraction best avoided!

to jot down the least clear point (sometimes called 'the muddiest point'), can be helpful in assessing intermittent understanding. Another method involves selecting a small focus group (perhaps including two learners each from the high, middle and low performing thirds). This group might respond to pre-identified quality prompts and could be facilitated by a postgraduate student or another informed person who is not directly involved with the course.

The advent of technology has allowed for increased access to just-in-time (yet still semi-anonymous) collection of data as well as learner-initiated public review sites (see Box 5.3). For example, courseware such as Moodle and Blackboard includes polling functions that allow a teacher to ask content- and process-related questions in online survey format, receiving the responses instantly and with a variety of functions for reporting these data (e.g. bar charts). Although in most cases teachers can tell which learners have responded to the survey, they cannot link responses to individual learners.

Regardless of the method(s) selected, to obtain the best results, sufficient time must be devoted in advance to describing the review process to learners, assuring them that their feedback will not lead to reprisal and explaining how the information will be used for quality improvement.

Peers

A final source of opinion-based feedback on teaching effectiveness can come from peer evaluations. It may be the case at your institution that **peer evaluation** (or peer assessment) will be part of a standard probationary review for a new member of academic staff. In this case, a senior staff member will likely review your preparatory materials and attend a lecture or two. If there is no formal peer review process at your institution, it is appropriate to request this type of feedback. In either case, peer review can be a stressful process for both the evaluator and the evaluated, so care should be taken that the process (and implications) are clear to all involved.

When scientists submit an abstract for a conference or a bid for a research grant, these items undergo peer review. But while such peer review

Box 5.4 *Characteristics of an effective peer review process*

- It provides for both formative feedback and summative decision-making.
- The process and instrumentation have been developed with attention to thoroughness and fairness.
- Peer reviewers understand their task and are well prepared to accomplish it.
- Ongoing efforts in the academic unit are invested in improving the peer review process.
- Peer review assignments are made in ways that are likely to result in helpful collaborations.
- Peer review is a valued process within the academic unit.
- Parties are cooperative and timely in accomplishing peer review tasks.

processes have become accepted as standards in the academic community, peer review of teaching (a highly personal activity) still feels somewhat strange. Some teachers may see it as a violation of privacy, a lack of professional courtesy, or even a breach of egalitarianism in the classroom.

However, peer review of teaching is a professional responsibility that is vital to professional development and teaching excellence for both the full-time educator and the clinician/teacher. The key to helping staff feel more comfortable with the process is for there to be clarity about goals and procedures, with an emphasis placed on practicality and fairness (see Box 5.4).

To help prepare for formal peer review sessions, it may also be beneficial to hold informal review sessions with junior colleagues or mid-level staff. This can be an unstructured session, using a standardised form or a form customised to the specific course or discipline being evaluated. For one example of a peer lecture evaluation, see Appendix 8.

If your course objectives include building foundational knowledge to be used in future courses (e.g. a physiology course in preparation for a patho-physiology course) then you might consider seeking less direct (but also less intimidating) peer review. This can be achieved by asking the teacher of the subsequent course his perceptions of how prepared the learners were for the new content area. Clearly, your performance is only one factor that can influence this, but asking the question may identify any critical problems and can also open the door for future communications about how your content areas may be better linked.

Facts

Until this point, we have focused on a variety of opinions that may be useful in evaluating your teaching; so let us move on to a discussion of the facts. Facts may be collected from a variety of sources but the three that we will discuss are: examination performance statistics, video (recorded) files, and learning experts.

Examination performance statistics

As discussed in Chapter 4, creating sound assessments is a skill that must be developed by teachers. With regard to this, however, the teacher may not be working in isolation as both internal and external review or moderation of assessments is usual practice in many programmes. The good news is that in addition to revealing how much your learners know about a particular subject area, a sound assessment also provides an indirect measure of your teaching effectiveness. Note that this does not mean that a high average examination score is equivalent to good teaching; rather, that specifics about how well learners perform on individual items (or groups of items) may provide clues that contribute to a comprehensive review of teaching performance.

Specifically, when reviewing results from objective-style examinations (e.g. those consisting of multiple choice questions), techniques called **test-item analyses** (already mentioned in Chapter 4) can reveal which items:

1 Are more/less difficult
2 Best discriminate between high and low (overall) performing learners.

As discussed previously, test-item analysis judges each item against pre-defined external criteria or against the remaining items in the assessment. As a result, in addition to providing data for potential score adjustment at the learner level, such analyses can also be employed to revise and improve teaching and assessment skills.

Some universities may have centralised examination services that provide machine marking of objective examinations and produce these types of analyses. Even without such support, however, they are relatively straight-forward to do using a basic spreadsheet program (e.g. Microsoft Excel).

A complete description of the possible approaches utilised in test-item analysis is beyond the scope of this text; however, Box 5.5 includes a summary of the some of the key definitions and Davis (1993) provides more detail about this important tool.

Video files

Video-recording your teaching session, via a variety of media formats, is a very powerful tool for teaching improvement. If you have ready access

> *Box 5.5* *Key concepts in test-item analysis*
>
> **Difficulty**
>
> - The proportion of test takers who answered the question *incorrectly* varies between 0 and 1. The higher the proportion of wrong answerers, the greater the difficulty of the item.
> - If the purpose of a test is to discriminate between different levels of achievement, the optimal level of difficulty is 0.5.
>
> **Discrimination**
>
> - Discrimination relates to the ability of a question to distinguish between individuals who have a high overall score on the test (well prepared) and those who receive a relatively low score (less well prepared).
> - There are several measures of discrimination available; these are all influenced by the degree of difficulty of the item. Examples include:
>
>   o Extreme groups method
>   o Reliability indices

to institutional or personal recording equipment, it can also be one of the most cost-effective evaluation methods. Despite this you should accept that, for many, this can be a very awkward process, perhaps even more uncomfortable than peer review (see Personal view 5.1). Still, for the hardy, it is a very powerful tool at all levels of teaching, from the novice to the master.

Some programmes may have a formal video-recording procedure, particularly for new teachers, which involves creating and submitting media files to demonstrate competence in the classroom. If this is the case at your institution, you may choose to hold a few practice sessions to ensure you feel comfortable in front of the camera. You should also make sure that it is clear to learners that the recording process is a way to review *your* performance, not *theirs*. In some cases, it may also be prudent to clear the recording process with your programme's ethics review panel, to clarify that this is part of continuous quality improvement (and not research).

If your programme does not have a formal video-recording process, there may still be resources on the campus or in the community you can access, for example a media office or a journalism or theatre programme may have equipment and personnel trained for this task. If all else fails, a personal

Personal view 5.1

The first time I watched myself teach on videotape, I was absolutely mortified. The regional accent in my voice sounded so thick; my gestures were uncoordinated and distracting; and I seldom paused from speaking long enough for a learner to actually respond to one of the hours of preparation I had put into developing a meaningful lecture!

After the initial shock had passed, I reviewed the tape again … this time concentrating on the strengths as well as the areas for improvement. In retrospect, I had spent so much time worrying about mastering the scientific content – afraid that the learners would discover even a single fact about which I was unsure – that I had neglected to focus on the methods for communicating this information.

I then swallowed my pride and asked a mentor to review it with me. I shed a few tears but we laughed even more … and together we worked on a plan to help me synchronise my desire to be a good teacher with my skill in the classroom.

I didn't erase this tape for many years; instead I shared it with my own teaching mentees who were (thankfully) amazed at how much I had improved over time.

Brad, clinical lecturer

video camera placed on a tripod at the back of the classroom or other teaching setting may also work.

Some argue that knowing that your lecture is being recorded likely changes your teaching behaviour; however, experts agree that despite feeling uncomfortable at the beginning of the taping, this awkwardness resolves quickly and, owing to the complexity of the task and the nature of your responsibility to the learners, you quickly return to your natural instructional state.

Once you have recorded the lecture (if possible, capturing both your teaching behaviours and the learner reactions and interactions), find a private place to scan through it quickly; focusing first just on overall impressions. Be aware that the first things that typically jump out are details of appearance that, in reality, are likely more distracting on the tape than in real life.

After writing down your initial impressions, go through the tape once again but more slowly. On this viewing, focus on *measurable behaviours*, such as the frequencies and types of interactions between you and the learners (for example, how many queries requested a response from learners? Was sufficient time allowed for learner responses?). Some teachers find it helpful to use standard checklists to focus their analysis; others create tailored versions to reflect a specific area of interest or need.

Remember that reviewing a recorded lecture is one of the few ways to experience the class as the learners do – by viewing and listening as a third party. You can also examine the learners' responses to your teaching (which you may not be able to do at the same time as giving the lecture/facilitating the activity itself).

So, as uncomfortable as it may feel at first, you should take advantage of the opportunity to walk in the shoes of a learner.

Learning experts

A final source of fact-based feedback on teaching effectiveness can come from learning experts, who can be distinguished from peer reviewers because typically:

1 They do not come from a similar scientific discipline (e.g. healthcare)
2 They use educational theory to guide their reviews.

Note, however, that this traditional concept of learning expert is changing and, as health profession educators have begun exploring more innovative instructional methods, there have been some investments in developing expertise in medical education with particular emphasis on clinical sciences.

Because healthcare is ever changing, the ability to self-direct learning is rapidly being recognised as a critical skill and the ability to teach this skill is a lesson that also must be taught. The value of having a dedicated educational expert is that they can introduce or augment your knowledge of theory-based methods in teaching. When partnered with a content expert (such as a mentor within your discipline or school), this can be a very rich resource for new teachers or teachers looking to improve their performance.

Some programmes may have a centre for teaching and learning available specifically to assist teachers in developing their skills. In this case, there will likely be dedicated staff to provide not only feedback but also assistance in reviewing teaching activities and even developing assessments.

If your programme does not have a centre dedicated to teacher development, then consider seeking assistance from a school of education or a local teacher training programme.

How can you use these opinions and facts to redesign your course or teaching materials?

So far, this chapter has focused on a variety of opinion-based and fact-based sources of information for evaluating your teaching. The next step is using

Box 5.6   Beginning with the end

One good approach is to create a table of the major learner criticisms from the previous term along with how you as the teacher have addressed this for the next offering. This can then be distributed to, and discussed with, the current learners.

For example, if lectures ran long in the past, you might say that you have appointed a student timekeeper to remind you when there is five minutes left in the class. Even when a prior criticism has not been addressed, it is a good idea to reveal this. In the case that this is due to policy, you should state this clearly so that learners know that you did not have the authority to make this change. In the case that you don't have a viable solution, invite the current class to help with the improvement process.

By 'beginning with the end', learners see that you take their feedback seriously and will likely contribute more of their own suggestions.

this information to redesign your course, lecture or activity. With this in mind, it is important to consider:

- What *can* be changed quickly (e.g. add more review sessions)
- What *must wait* until the next time the course is offered (e.g. the textbook)
- What *cannot* or *will not* be changed (e.g. the course marking scheme).

Some interventions, such as learning to feel more comfortable speaking in front of a group, may take additional study or review. Others, such as adding page numbers to the course syllabus, may involve administrative assistance.

Creating a table of challenges and a plan to address these is an important way forward. To help focus your plan, look back to Chapter 2 to get some ideas on redesigning your teaching material, and Chapter 3 for tips on how to improve the delivery of your course.

The most important thing to remember about using evaluation to re-design a course or activity is that it is always best to be honest about your goals (see Box 5.6). This will also help to ensure that your methods stay aligned with your teaching philosophy.

Why do both teachers and learners often resist the improvement process?

Evaluating and redesigning teaching can be a time-consuming process and time is the most valuable asset of a teacher; particularly for those who also

Box 5.7 *Resistance to change*

Misguided teachers often explain disappointing teaching evaluations by *externalising* the blame. Some of these reasons include:

- Unmotivated learners
- Vindictive peers
- Heavy teaching loads
- Invalid rating systems.

One can imagine that such teachers have approached learning in the same way that they were taught (with a heavy focus on passive lecture and only minimal student interaction). This *known* approach feels comfortable so it continues despite a lack of effectiveness.

Just as the science of our respective health disciplines changes over time, so do the learners, the learning environment and the learning process itself.

Clinicians would agree that scientific discovery has yielded a greater number and higher quality of targeted medicines with which to treat diseases today compared with even ten years ago. Likewise, there are more and better methods for approaching teaching. For this reason, our teaching must be just as dynamic and innovative as the sciences we represent. Good teachers accept responsibility for ensuring that this occurs.

have clinical and research activities to support. All new teaching methods (just like new scientific methods) involve some degree of risk and some of us are naturally more averse to this risk than others. Box 5.7 includes some of the common excuses for poor results, but, in truth, the root cause for this resistance to innovation is usually fear.

Teachers are typically acutely aware that poor learner, peer and expert reviews make them very vulnerable to organisational reprimand. This can manifest as fear of resistance to new teaching methods. In addition, some teachers fear that by introducing more interactive learning strategies (such as those described in Chapter 3), they will lose time for 'content coverage' especially in foundational courses.

In response to these arguments, we advise that when pedagogy is founded in evidence-based methods and includes self-reflection and peer review, then some resistance (especially initially) will not likely be reason enough to draw organisational concern. As for the loss of content coverage time, careful monitoring and documentation will ensure that learner outcomes from more engaging strategies are just as high as (or even higher than) with traditional lecture.

Some teachers incorrectly assume that learners prefer passive methods, but in reality this is often a function of time. Educational policies may base the amount of permissible **contact hours** on the traditional lecture model whereby learners complete most of the learning time within the confines of the classroom. If the teacher suddenly shifts to a **self-directed learning** model, this may impact on how much time the learner has to study and reflect, especially in the case of multiple classes being taken concomitantly (as described in Chapter 2). If this is suspected to be the issue, consider using the course evaluation process to probe for potential solutions with learners and with peers.

What should you do with the products of the teaching evaluation process once you have used them to improve your teaching?

Some teachers think that once a self-reflection, learner survey, peer review, or video file has been reviewed and the respective changes to a course have been made, these tools have served their purpose and can be discarded. But as mentioned previously, the sheer volume of material about teaching sessions, assessments and learners means that specifics will fade over time and yet these same details are invaluable for decision-making in the future. Most importantly, spiral reflection on these issues (see Chapter 6), delving ever deeper as you gain more experience, can feed back into the process for refining your teaching philosophy (see Chapter 1).

Increasingly, education experts suggest that including excerpts or summaries of this same information as part of a teaching portfolio is a very rich way to monitor change in teaching effectiveness over time. A teaching portfolio is a document that describes how we collect, analyse, interpret, and use data to modify or improve teaching. Some academic programmes are requiring these tools as part of the hiring or promotion process; for others, they are used more informally.

It is beyond the scope of this chapter to include a detailed discussion of teaching portfolios, but Seldin *et al.* (2006) can be reviewed for more information about this tool.

Summary

The motivation to improve your teaching practices based on experience, review and reflection is affected by both intrinsic and extrinsic factors. Teachers who care about learning tend to try harder and longer to improve their skills, but it does not mean that the pathway is any easier.

In fact, the motivated but inexperienced teacher can sometimes become disheartened by even one poor evaluation. Just as we started this chapter by stating that it is reasonable that not every teaching session will yield the intended results, it is also reasonable that despite your best efforts there will still be someone who is not completely satisfied for reasons that may or may not be related to the teacher's skill.

When considering your evaluations holistically, we advise that you:

- Consider the balance of negative comments compared with positive comments
- Do not take negativity as a personal attack
- Try to find the kernel of truth within any complaint; focusing only on this aspect to improve your teaching.

Remember that by evaluating your teaching and redesigning your courses, lectures, activities and assessments on the basis of the opinions and facts you have collected and analysed, you are *learning about learning* at the same time as you are *teaching* learners about the knowledge, skills and attitudes associated with a specific content area. Modelling these lifelong learning skills may actually be the best educational intervention you can ever make.

Top tips

- Explore the teaching evaluation resources available through your department, school, university, hospital or other clinical practice site. Often there are designated experts who can assist you with evaluating and improving your teaching. If there is no formal Teaching & Learning Office, consider the schools or departments of education or communication.
- After reviewing any annual teaching evaluation requirements required by your programme, map out a comprehensive teaching evaluation plan with your department head or line manager. This is a good way to informally assess the degree of organisational support you will have for teaching. Even if this is low, your supervisor will likely appreciate the systematic approach and it will minimise the risk of unpleasant surprises later.
- Identify a teaching mentor or mentors (within your school or discipline or from an external group). If you do not know anyone, ask learners who the 'best' teachers are in the programme. This information will be subjective, but it can guide you to open a conversation with other staff. Ask to sit in on one of their lectures, discuss your evaluation plan, or ask them for an informal peer review.

- Start or join a 'better teaching' peer group. This can be a group of staff from your own programme that meets informally or even an online community of academic or clinical staff you meet through training or professional meetings.

References and further reading

Boyer E (1990). *Scholarship Reconsidered: Priorities for the Professoriate*. Princeton, NJ: Carnegie Foundation for the Advancement of Teaching.

Breslow L, Schuster JM (2007). Problems, pitfalls and surprises in teaching: Mini cases. In: Ross C *et al.*, eds. *Strategies for Teaching Assistant and International Teaching Assistant Development: Beyond Micro Teaching*. San Francisco, CA: Jossey-Bass.

Chism NV (2007). Why introducing or sustaining peer review of teaching is so hard and what you can do about it. *The Department Chair: A Resource for Academic Administrators* 18(2; Fall).

Chism NV (2007). Setting up a system of peer review. *Peer Review of Teaching: A Sourcebook*. San Francisco, CA: Jossey-Bass.

Davis BG (1993). *Tools for Teaching*. San Francisco, CA: Jossey-Bass.

Deselle SP, Hammer DP (2002). *Handbook for Pharmacy Education: Getting Adjusted as a New Faculty Member*. Binghamton, NY: The Haworth Press.

Gronlund NE, Linn RL (1990). *Measurement and Evaluation in Teaching*, 6th edn. New York: Macmillan.

Hodges LC (2006). Helping faculty deal with fear. In: *To Improve the Academy, Resources for Faculty, Instructional and Organizational Development*, Vol. 24. San Francisco, CA: Jossey-Bass.

Hoyt DP, Pallett WH (1999). *Appraising Teaching Effectiveness: Beyond Student Ratings*. IDEA Paper #36. Manhatan, KS: The Idea Center, www.theideacenter.org/category/helpful-resources/knowledge-base/idea-papers (accessed 27 February 2011).

Lee D, Sabatino K (1998). Evaluating guided reflections: a US case study. *International Journal of Training and Development* 2(3): 162–170.

Lucas AF (2002). Reaching the unreachable: improving the teaching of poor teachers. In: *A Guide to Faculty Development Practical Advice, Examples, and Resources*. Professional and Organizational Development Network in Higher Education. San Francisco, CA: Anker/Jossey-Bass.

McKeachie WJ (1999). *McKeachie's Teaching Tips: Strategies, Research, and Theory for College and University Teachers*. Boston, MA: Houghton Mifflin.

Rhem J (2006). The high risks of improving teaching. TP Msg# 760. Tomorrow's Professor Mailing List.

Seldin P (2004). *The Teaching Portfolio: A Practical Guide to Improved Performance and Promotion/Tenure Decisions*, 3rd ed. Boston, MA: Anker.

Seldin P *et al.* (2006). Uses and abuses of student ratings. In: *Evaluating Faculty Performance: A Practical Guide to Assessing Teaching, Research, and Service*. San Francisco, CA: Anker/Jossey-Bass.

Resources

This is an excellent (and free) resource covering a large range of topics associated with learning and evaluation. The site is not specific to health professions education, although many clinical examples are given. Weekly messages, usually extracted from current literature or professional discussions, can be sent directly to your email or you can access them from the website. www.stanford.edu/dept/CTL/Tomprof/index.shtml (accessed 9 March 2011).

AACP Education Scholar is designed for the busy professional, and offers a comprehensive online curriculum that will expand your knowledge and skills as a health professions teacher. Module concepts are presented through a combination of on-screen text, images and audio clips. Examples, case studies and demonstrations from the health professions are included to illustrate key points. This comprehensive resource is focused on developing stronger teachers in the field of pharmacy, although most of the information would apply to any health professions training program. There is a fee associated with accessing the materials, but it could be used by an individual or a group (e.g. a department) for a team-based approach. www.aacp.org/CAREER/EDUCATIONSCHOLAR/Pages/default. aspx (accessed 9 March 2011).

6

Reflecting on teaching and learning

Sue C Jones and Barry Jubraj

Developing skills and improving performance are vital in any profession. You have already been introduced to the concept of reflection earlier in the book. Reflection is a process that allows you to consider your skills and performance, and develop ways to improve and enhance your practice. This chapter will help you to understand what reflection is, why it is important, and how to do it. We explain how thinking critically about your practice as a teacher can develop your teaching skills, thereby making you more effective at improving your students' learning. Regardless of your existing profession or job, this chapter will show you how to draw on your personal experiences in order to inform your teaching role.

This chapter contains some exercises that aim to help you apply what you have read to your own situation. When answering the questions, go with your gut responses. It might also be helpful to jot down your thoughts – make a note of any changes you would like to make to your teaching practice and any ideas for improvements.

'Reflection' – a dirty word?

It may be tempting to skip over a chapter on 'reflection' if you are not fully aware of the concept or do not understand its importance. (See Personal view 6.1 for one experience.) It can be perceived as a 'touchy-feely' subject, or less relevant than other evaluation strategies. In addition, students with science backgrounds may find it unfamiliar and uncomfortable, and they can be particularly poor at expressing themselves in writing (Gibbs 1988).

Professionals in all fields think about what they are doing, respond to feedback and make changes for the future. In other words, they reflect.

What is reflection and why do it?

In simple terms, reflection is thinking about one's experiences. Chapter 5 explained methods of evaluating one's teaching by seeking the opinions

Personal view 6.1

When I first heard about reflection I didn't really know what it meant or how to do it. But my colleague told me that an easy way to start was to ask myself a few questions after I had done something:

- What went well?
- What didn't go so well?
- If I did it again what would I change?
- If I did it again what would I leave the same?

This really helped me think more objectively about my activities. When I came to teach for the first time I found I was able to reflect on the lesson and make changes to improve it for the next time.

Adebayo, pharmacist

of others – peers, mentors and learners themselves. Reflection is a way to self-evaluate one's teaching.

Reflective practice encourages teachers to think critically about the principles and practices underlying their work, and to be prepared to change or modify their teaching in response to feedback. It can encourage and support teachers to make use of peer review and students' feedback, and to think about the efficiency and effectiveness of their teaching strategies.

Reflection also enables teachers to learn from their teaching experiences. It is worth noting that there are often consequences of not being reflective, such as teaching out-of-date information.

Learning to reflect

Using your own experience is one of the best ways to improve. Reflection can help you to learn from your successes, as well as from your mistakes. By reflecting on previous experiences you can plan for similar situations in the future, and decide on what worked and what to do differently.

How to get started

Many people when they try to reflect find it very hard to get going, let alone to come up with anything useful. These exercises may help get you started:

1 What comes to your mind when you think of the word 'reflection'?
2 When do you have your greatest ideas? At a certain time of day? Or when you are doing a particular activity such as walking to work or lying in bed?

Personal view 6.2

A leading authority on diabetes was invited to deliver a lecture to my class. At the end of the lecture I couldn't wait to moan to other students about the lecturer seeming disengaged, exemplified by him pacing up and down in front of the presentation and not making eye contact with any of us. The lecturer therefore didn't see the occasional raised hand for questions and didn't notice our lack of understanding of what he was saying. As a consequence of him being a leading authority, he gave the impression that the purpose of the session was to give a lecture on 'everything I know about diabetes'.

Some weeks later, we had a stand-in lecturer, covering sickness. At the start, the lecturer acknowledged that he was not an expert on the topic, and told us that this had made him research and try to understand the principles for himself. At the end of the lecture, there was a real buzz in the lecture theatre, and when the lecturer left after taking questions, we couldn't stop talking about how clear and helpful the lecture had been. We really noticed his approachability in the lecture and his enthusiasm for our learning was obvious.

Paul, medical undergraduate

3 If you have had a previous teaching experience did you think about it afterwards? Did you look through the evaluation forms immediately? Did you focus on the positive or the negative comments?

4 Do you ever have useful thoughts about your work that you subsequently forget? Can you think of ways to record them for reflection later on? Some people keep a notebook with them or email themselves a message. What might work for you?

Professional identity

Some individuals who are new to teaching in healthcare may come from a professional or vocational background. As such, they will be experienced as, say, clinical practitioners yet as new teachers they will be moving out of their comfort zone. It is important not to assume that an expert in the field will automatically be an effective teacher (see Personal view 6.2).

A small identity crisis can occur as you develop an educational role while maintaining or even moving away from your original profession. For some teachers in healthcare the balance may shift so that they begin to view themselves primarily as educators. One way to spot this is to look at your

Personal view 6.3

Part of my current role involves me helping my colleagues to record their continuing professional development (CPD). One of my team, Namita, was finding this particularly difficult. She had been qualified in her profession for many years and was the expert in her field. She felt that there was little room for improvement. While I was chatting with her, Namita told me that she regularly helps with her son's football team and recently took a football coaching course. As we were talking she realised that she had used some of the skills she had learnt on the football coaching course and applied them at work. These new skills had helped her in her clinical practice and in dealing with staffing issues and in particular dealing with conflict.

I realised that experiences and skills learnt in our spare time can also be useful when applied at work.

Kaaria, nurse

continuing professional development (CPD) records. What is the balance of your records? Do more of them cover teaching and training rather than your original profession?

It is not a problem if the balance shifts, but it can be a valuable prompt for reflection on the balance of your professional responsibilities. Teachers in healthcare need to maintain their development in both teaching and their professional practice.

A shift in roles may also be accompanied by a shift in perceptions. As you move towards an academic role in teaching, training or tutoring others, you may be perceived differently by yourself and others, including your patients, clients, colleagues or students. We suggest that you regularly review how up-to-date you are in your profession as you balance your responsibilities.

You can also take advantage of your dual identity. For example, if you are a chemist, your talent for accuracy and precision can help ensure that you plan your teaching sessions thoroughly. If you are a clinical practitioner, think about how your 'duty of care' as a clinician can be transferred to those you teach.

If you find yourself struggling to reconcile your two distinct roles, try asking yourself who you think you are, primarily, as a professional. Are you comfortable with your answer? Why might you feel that way? You might also consider finding someone else in your situation to see whether they have any helpful insights for you (see Personal view 6.3).

Reflecting on your role as a teacher in the healthcare professions

Whatever your profession, your experience will differ from the experience of others whose primary professional training was as a teacher. Your perceptions of teaching may also be different from those of others.

For example, some teachers in healthcare may attach less importance to the underpinning educational theory than those whose initial professional training was as a teacher. In addition, some teachers in healthcare may teach primarily from their own experience, which can differ between individuals. Some may feel the pressure of having to keep up-to-date in both their professional role and their job as a teacher.

As such, there are potential pitfalls for the new teacher in healthcare, and it is important to think about how you arrived in this dual role, and your motivations, perceptions and concerns.

Your teaching role

Consider how you feel about teaching as a role, how you perform as a teacher, and how you might be perceived as a teacher.

1 What is the greatest reward you get from teaching?
2 What is your greatest fear when you teach?
3 Is there something that you could change about your teaching to maximise the reward or minimise the fear?
4 Some say that the best person to teach is an expert. Others disagree. What do you think about these views and why?
5 List some of the words or phrases that you think your students or colleagues would use to describe you as a teacher. Now compare these words and phrases with the evaluations you have actually had of your teaching. Are your perceptions similar to those of your students?

Competence in reflective practice as a teacher in healthcare

Competency (or professional development) frameworks have been developed in the UK's National Health Service (NHS) to describe the knowledge, skills, values and attitudes required for professional practice. According to the Competency Development and Evaluation Group (CoDEG), **competence** is 'the ability to carry out a job or task'. A **competency** is 'a quality or characteristic of a person related to effective or superior performance'. It is made up of many things such as knowledge, skills, attitudes and traits.

But as a new teacher it can be quite difficult to judge how good or competent you are unless someone or something encourages you to reflect, learn and change.

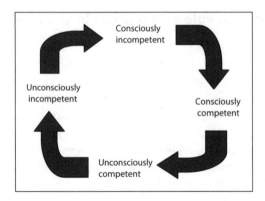

Figure 6.1. May and Kruger's competence cycle. (Adapted from May and Kruger (1988).)

May and Kruger (1988) suggested that competence involves a cycle like that shown in Fig. 6.1.

Let us use an example. You have been asked to teach professional ethics to a group of healthcare professionals that includes undergraduate medical, nursing and pharmacy students. As you are only aware of your own professional code of ethics, you feel very much out of your depth. At this moment you are conscious that you do not know enough; you are *consciously incompetent*.

You decide that the best way to prepare for this session would be to do some research about the various healthcare professional codes of ethics and set up some group work for the students. You find out about the similarities and differences between the professional groups you are teaching and work out how you will plan your session.

Feeling more confident you will have moved around the cycle to *consciously competent*. You then run the session and reflect on how the session went. This includes your own reflections, student evaluations, and anecdotal comments from students after the session.

When you are asked to run the session the following year you may still be in the *consciously competent* phase. But once you have repeatedly run the session, you may move to the *unconsciously competent* phase. You know what you are teaching in depth and you are able to teach it almost instinctively without considering consciously how you are doing it.

This may carry on for many years. However, you neglect to update your handouts and materials and your students notice that you are a bit out-of-date as some of their codes of ethics have changed. In this scenario you are unaware of the limitations of your teaching and are *unconsciously incompetent*. This may or may not continue unless one of your students questions your information.

You start to worry and question your ability to teach and your teaching materials. You are *consciously incompetent* and the cycle begins again.

Being 'good enough'

It may be helpful to mention perfectionism here, which some health professionals may exhibit. If you have a tendency towards perfectionism, this characteristic may manifest itself as you gain experience in planning and delivering teaching. Learning to be 'good enough', as the paediatrician and psychiatrist Donald Winnicott encouraged, can be preferable to unhealthily striving for perfection that may not be possible.

Your own level of competence

Have a think about your own competence by answering the questions below. You can think about experiences from your professional life or your personal life.

1 Think about a time when you last felt consciously incompetent about something. How did you feel? Were you calm or did you panic? Did you have any physical signs of nervousness?
2 Think about the last time you learned something new. How did it feel to be conscious of your newly acquired skill, knowledge or behaviour? Were you confident?
3 Have you ever had the feeling that the person talking to you didn't really know what they were talking about? Why did you think this? Have you ever been in a similar situation where you were very unsure of the information you were giving out? How did you feel?

The 'Competence versus Confidence model'

Teaching with confidence is vital for your own well-being and development as a teacher, as well as for ensuring that your students can trust the information you give them, with all the attendant consequences for patient care. Even if you are unsure about something, communicating this honestly and confidently will lead to trust and respect.

Fig. 6.2 shows the Competence versus Confidence model. This may help you if it feels like the confidence and competence you developed through your original profession have deserted you as you begin your role as a teacher.

The model can help you understand the relationship between confidence and competence in addition to providing you with insight into the changes you may experience when learning how to teach, and helping you reflect on your progress.

You may also be able to think back to your development in your original profession. Were you confident as you entered your profession or did you lack self-belief? Consider how your confidence changed as you

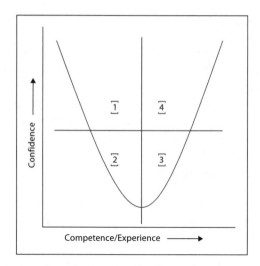

Figure 6.2. The Competence versus Confidence model. (Model adapted with permission by London Pharmacy Education and Training from the Situational Leadership II Model by Hersey and Blanchard. (See Changing Minds.org (2011).)

developed skills, demonstrated your competence, or suffered setbacks. (See Personal view 6.4.)

This model shows four quadrants. You will see that in quadrant 1, the individual's competence and experience are low but confidence is high. Initially, your professional expertise may make you confident, but as a new teacher you have little experience and competence in teaching. Don't worry if your confidence is not high initially.

In quadrant 2, confidence has dropped, perhaps with early experience and setbacks; but competence has increased due to that experience. As time goes on, experience increases along with competence, and subsequently your confidence grows (quadrant 3). 'Peak performance' is shown in quadrant 4, where both confidence and competence are high.

The Confidence versus Competence model can also help you identify, perhaps with help from someone you trust, whether and when you need support in your new role. At the start of their training experience (e.g. quadrants 1 and 2) new teachers may require supervision and support when they are unsure of what to do, what is expected of them or how to carry out their roles and responsibilities.

Remember that you will have previously developed your confidence and competence in your previous roles. You are likely to need to repeat the process as a teacher.

Personal development

Having read this chapter, try the following exercises to help you think about your next steps.

Personal view 6.4

I was asked to deliver a talk to about 90 pre-registration pharmacy graduates when I was a relatively junior practitioner. Their conduct during the talk was very poor, and may have partly resulted from my inexperience. I left the session demoralised and with my confidence low.

The next year I asked if I could do the session again, as I was determined to overcome this difficulty. I decided on a strategy: I had a list of all the graduates' names and had thought of questions that I could ask periodically throughout the session. I was careful to make the questions opinion-based rather than asking for information that they might get wrong and feel threatened by. I wasn't worried about knowing the person I decided to call out to; I just looked out confidently at the lecture theatre.

The effect was striking. There was a mixture of attentiveness, and possibly nervousness about being asked for an opinion; but those asked seemed happy to answer. I reflected afterwards that I had gained some confidence in how to manage a large group by trying out something like this. Since then, I am happy to use this strategy again and have developed the effectiveness of it so that I can stimulate discussion and reflection in large groups.

Rafal, pharmacist

1 Think about your strengths and areas for development. What do you think you are 'good enough' at? What aspects of teaching do you need to improve?
2 What changes, if any, are you going to make?
3 Could you use your professional development obligations to help you develop as a teacher, and vice versa?

Summary

If you are not used to it, reflecting on your teaching may be difficult at first. However, it is fundamentally important and relevant to your development as a new teacher. The exercises will have encouraged you to reflect on your personal skills, your new role as a teacher, and your teaching experiences so far. The insight you gain into your performance as a teacher will enable you to improve and achieve, and will ultimately benefit your students.

Top tips

- If you are not used to reflecting, start simply. Reflect on something you did today. Just get started.
- Don't forget to focus on the positive aspects, not just the negative – what went well today?
- As well as taking the time to reflect alone, remember that you can also reflect with others in your team – discussion with your peers, your boss, your staff and your other stakeholders can provide very useful insights.
- Do not assume that because you know your subject well, you can teach it well. Always be prepared to improve.

References and further reading

Changing Minds.org (2011). *Hersey and Blanchard's Situational Leadership.* http://changingminds.org/disciplines/leadership/styles/situational_leadership_hersey_blanchard.htm (accessed 11 March 2011).

Gibbs G (1988). *Learning by Doing: A Guide to Teaching and Learning Methods.* Oxford: Further Education Unit, Oxford Brookes University; 96.

May GD, Kruger M (1988). The manager within. *Personnel Journal* 67(2): 57–65.

Morris K *et al.* (2010). Make reflection part of your daily practice. *Clinical Pharmacist* 2: 397–399.

Moon JA (2004). *Reflection in Learning and Professional Development: Theory and Practice.* London: RoutledgeFalmer.

Schon DA (1990). *Educating the Reflective Practitioner: Toward a New Design for Teaching and Learning.* London: Jossey-Bass.

Schon DA (1991). *The Reflective Practitioner: How Professionals Think in Action.* London: Ashgate.

Steiner ID (1972). *Group Process and Productivity.* New York: Academic Press.

For more information on professional development frameworks

www.codeg.org.

The Hersey and Blanchard Situational Leadership II Model

http://plaza.ufl.edu/normans/AS300%20Lsn%2018%20SitLead.ppt.

For pharmacy education and training

www.londonpharmacy.nhs.uk/EducationAndTraining/index.aspx.

Appendix 1

Tips for overcoming challenges related to teaching in your healthcare practice site

1 Help students feel that they belong in the practice site

- Be friendly and patient.
- Include students in what you are doing.
- Be sensitive to issues related to age, culture, gender, ethnicity, and religious beliefs.
- Introduce students to others in the work site.
- Encourage students to interact with you and others, as appropriate.

2 Orient students to the practice site

- Be prepared and organised.
- Clearly communicate your expectations to students.
- Ask students for their goals and expectations for learning.
- Tour the physical facilities.
- Review the schedule, appropriate dress, policies, etc.
- Clarify how the students' learning will be evaluated.
- Ask students for their expectations of you.
- Let students know who they will interact with and in what way.
- Encourage students to take an active role in their learning.
- Help students to identify a realistic, appropriate amount of time or effort to spend on the various tasks and activities that you assign.
- Encourage students to challenge themselves and learn from their mistakes.

3 Use effective verbal and non-verbal communication

- Use good eye contact and positive facial expressions and body language.
- Be aware of students' unspoken emotions and that they may be fearful.
- Keep students informed of any changes in the rotation.
- Provide specific constructive feedback – let students know what they need to improve and how, and acknowledge all improvement.
- Try to adapt your teaching style to students' learning needs.

Source: Western University of Health Sciences and American Association of Colleges of Pharmacy (2010). *Education Scholar Module 4C: Learning in the Experiential Setting.* Available online at www.educationscholar.org (accessed 22 March 2010).

Appendix 2

Guide for developing your teaching philosophy

Your ultimate philosophy of teaching will be based upon your own thoughts about education, teaching and learning and on a combination of common sense, your own past learning experiences, and teaching theories. As you reflect on your philosophy over time, you are likely to refine it on the basis of your personal experiences and reflection.

However, to begin capturing your teaching philosophy in words, *reflect on the three major questions below*. You need not address all of the sub-questions – these are simply intended to help get you thinking.

1 What do I really believe about teaching and learning?

- What is my purpose and role as a teacher?
- What do I believe about teaching and learning methods, the learning environment, teacher responsibilities, student responsibilities, etc.?
- Why do I enjoy teaching or want to teach?
- What makes me feel good about my teaching?

2 What does my teaching look like now?

- Are my current beliefs about teaching and learning evident? Are they useful?
- What teaching methods do I use most often?
- Why do I use these teaching methods rather than others?
- What seems to work the best in my current approach to teaching? What doesn't work so well?

3 What do I want my teaching to look like in the future?

- What are my teaching goals?
- What do I want or need to change about how I teach in order to reach these goals?

- What learning outcomes do I want students to achieve as a result of my teaching?
- What do students need to know and do in my class order to achieve these outcomes?
- What are the best teaching methods to help students achieve these outcomes?
- How will I know when I have achieved my teaching goals?
- How will I know when my students have achieved the learning outcomes?

Sources: Center for Effective Teaching and Learning at the University of Texas at El Paso (CETaL). *Articulating Your Philosophy of Teaching.* http://sunconference.utep.edu/CETaL/resources/portfolios/writetps.htm# comments.

Chism NV (1997–1998). Developing a philosophy of teaching statement. *Essays on Teaching Excellence: Toward The Best in the Academy 9.3.*

Hobson EH, Waite NM (2007). *Articulating a Teaching Philosophy.* www. aacp.org/AAP2007HobsonTeachingPhilosophySessionHandout.pdf.

Western University of Health Sciences and American Association of Colleges of Pharmacy (2010). Education Scholar Module 1: Developing a Personal Working Philosophy to Guide Teaching/Learning in the Health Professions Education.

Appendix 3

Template lesson plan

Topic		Course			Name of teacher	
Day/Date	Duration/Time	Class/Group	Period		Venue	Number of students

Purpose

Know what you want the lesson to achieve. Start by making this clear to the learners.

Learning experiences

Divide the lesson up into segments in which sub-topics will be addressed. Decide on the best strategy, for example to explain or illustrate concepts, or how to encourage participation by students.

1

2

3

Resources

Identify what resources will be needed for each learning segment. This will depend on your teaching goals, what you plan to do and what you expect the students to do. For example, equipment for presentations, handouts prior to and during the teaching session for students.

Conclusion

This draws together the learning experiences from the lesson. It should provide a summary of what has been said or demonstrated and an indication of how it will be extended into the next lesson.

Observations

These are your notes about how the students responded to your teaching strategies in the lesson. They provide the basis on which you reflect on the positive and negative aspects of the course and plan improvements for the future.

Appendix 4

Example OSCE

This example is taken from a postgraduate pharmacy practice diploma OSCE (Joint Programmes Board 2009). There are three individuals involved in this OSCE: the learner, an actor (nurse in charge), and an assessor.

Information given to learner

Framing

Read the following information carefully. You have ten minutes to complete the task in full.

Task

You are on a busy medical ward when the nurse in charge approaches you holding a drug chart. He/she asks whether you can help with a problem. Make an appropriate recommendation, including providing details relating to drug administration. The doctor is not currently available. You may assume that the sliding scale insulin has been previously checked, is being administered through a dedicated IV site and is appropriate.

ADDITIONAL INFORMATION

MICROBIOLOGY RESULTS

Name: Ms Grace Keller   Unit No : 214967

D.O.B. 10th March 1963   Consultant: Mr Shahid

Ward A2

REPORT

Sample received from a swab taken from a leg ulcer on the patient's left leg demonstrates a moderate growth of staphylococci species.

The antibiotic sensitivities are as follows (S = sensitive; R = resistant):

ERYTHROMYCIN	S
FLUCLOXACILLIN	S
FUSIDIC ACID	S
CEFUROXIME	R
MUPIROCIN	S

SAMPLE DETAILS

Sample taken today and results sent to ward.

Information given to assessor/actor

Opening Comment

Mrs Keller is a diabetic lady with spreading cellulitis who has been prescribed intravenous erythromycin to treat her cellulitis and you need a supply of the drug and advice on how to administer it. The doctors are insistent that the patient should receive therapy via the IV route as she had previously been given two weeks of oral antibiotics by her GP (which didn't work).

Responses (if asked)

1 Renal function is normal/good.
2 Erythromycin is to be given through a peripheral line situated in the right forearm.
3 Patient is a diabetic, also currently receiving a sliding-scale dose of insulin through a cannula on her left hand.
4 Patient has cellulitis – probably from a foot ulcer. It is now spreading up her leg.
5 Patient allergic to penicillin (rash and swollen lips) but front of drug chart not completed.
6 Vein is patent and is flushed with sodium chloride 0.9%.
7 GP started oral antibiotics but the leg became worse after 2 weeks' oral therapy. Patient then admitted to hospital and doctors are insisting on IV therapy. Unclear what patient received from her GP – think it's cefradine 1 gram bd.
8 Swab from foot ulcer shows staph. species – sensitive to flucloxacillin, erythromycin and fusidic acid but resistant to

cephalosporins. You may show the attached micro report to the pharmacist.

9 Diluting volume for erythromycin = 100 mL (as stated on drug chart); infusion time is 10 minutes.

Assessor criteria

	Achieved	Not achieved
Task is completed in a professional manner		
Adopts a structured approach to the task		
Checks that erythromycin is appropriate for infection (sensitivities)		
Identifies that erythromycin concentration too high (volume insufficient)		
Identifies erythromycin infusion rate is too rapid		
Identifies patient allergic to penicillin		
Advises to dilute to at least 250 mL with sodium chloride 0.9%		
Advises to administer slowly over 20 to 60 min		
Advises nurse to monitor cannula site regularly and consider re-siting if necessary		
Suggests chart is endorsed with administration information		
Identifies fusidic acid as adjunct therapy with erythromycin if infection not responding		
Asks about regular prescribed medicines		

Assessor's Comments

Recommendation (tick most appropriate term):

Pass criteria: 8 out of 12 (essential: italics)

Fail ☐   Pass ☐

Source: Joint Programmes Board (2009). *Assessment Handbook.* London. www.jpbsoutheast.org/about/

Appendix 5

Sample self-evaluation of teaching

Self-evaluation of teaching can be based on an end-of term review of any daily or weekly teaching reflections that have been compiled or summarised.

Scale:

   1 = not at all
   2 = slightly
   3 = somewhat
   4 = completely

Item	Term 1	Term 2
Made learning objectives clear to students		
Knowledgeable in the subject area		
Well-prepared		
Able to communicate concepts effectively		
Stimulated interest in the subject		
Effectively encouraged student participation		
Overall effectiveness in teaching		

	Term 1	Term 2
Strengths		
Weaknesses		

Goals for next year: _____

Appendix 6

What one thing do you wish we had spent **more** time doing (so far) in the course this term?

What one thing do you wish we had spent **less** time doing (so far) in the course this term?

What concept or skill do you feel that you understand better because of this course?

What can we do to improve this course?

Would you like to have the opportunity to 'shadow' a health professional on ward rounds some time this year? If so, should this be a required or voluntary activity?

Your comments are an important part of the continuous quality improvement of this course. Thank you for taking the time to help make this a better learning experience for all of us.

Appendix 7

Sample end-of-term evaluation

Using the following scales, select one response for each statement that best represents your opinion about the course and the course coordinators:

Questions 1–9

1 = strongly disagree; 2 = disagree; 3 = not sure; 4 = agree; 5 = strongly agree

1. The course followed a logical organisation and sequence of topics.
2. Class discussion was encouraged in this course.
3. When needed, the student was able to get personal help in this course.
4. My grade in this course accurately reflects my achievement of the course goals and objectives.
5. The course increased my knowledge and/or competence in this area.
6. The course clarified topics that were previously not clear to me.
7. The course pack was helpful and well-organised.
8. When possible, the instructors were flexible to the needs expressed by the students.
9. The goals and objectives of this course were distributed to me in writing at the beginning of the semester.

Questions 10–15

1 = never; 2 = seldom; 3 = sometimes; 4 = often; 5 = always

10. The pharmaceutics material supported the achievement of the stated goals and objectives.
11. Recitation activities supported the achievement of the stated goals and objectives.
12. 'Hands-on activities' in the skills lab helped me to better understand concepts introduced to me in other courses in the curriculum.

13. Working as a part of a team was better than completing all the work independently.
14. The guidelines for preparation for examinations, lab exercises, and recitations were clear.
15. The course coordinators were accessible and willing to provide help or clarification when needed.

Questions 16–17

Use the scale included in the text of the question.

16. The amount of work required to prepare for Skills Lab was:
    far too little (1), about right (3), or excessive (5)
17. The time allotted to complete Skills Lab activities was:
    far too short (1), about right (3), or far too long (5)

Questions 18–23

Please rate each of the following in terms of how useful you think that experience will be to you in the future. Comments on why you feel this way would be appreciated.

1 = totally useless; 2 = of very little use; 3 = somewhat useful; 4 = very useful; 5 = essential

18. Counselling/discussions from Top 200 Medications
19. P&T monograph assignment
20. Professional portfolio
21. Preparation of suppositories
22. Physical assessment and monitoring (e.g. blood glucose, peak flow, pregnancy tests)
23. Drug literature evaluation assignments

Questions 24–28

Please provide written comments.

24. How useful did you find the course webpage?
25. The things I liked most about this course were:
26. The things I would suggest to improve this course are:
27. Areas on which I would like to focus next term:
28. Additional comments or observations:

Your comments are an important part of the continuous quality improvement of this course.

Thank you for taking the time to help make this a better learning experience for all of us.

Appendix 8

Sample peer review of teaching checklist

Teacher Observed: _____ Course/Lecture: _____

Peer Reviewer: _____ Date: _____

Consider each element below and evaluate the teaching skills of the teacher by placing a check mark under the term best describing your evaluation of the teacher's actions. Add comments to illustrate your evaluation. Provide at least a summary evaluation in each category and details on individual points where you feel you have observed enough to make them.

Class organisation

The teacher:	Needs improvement	Effective	Highly effective	Not applicable	Comments
Started class on time					
Introduced lesson (overview or focusing activity)					
Paced topics appropriately					
Sequenced topics logically					
Related lesson to previous or future lessons or assignments					
Summarised or reviewed major lesson points					
Ended class on time					
Summary					

Presentation

The teacher:	Needs improvement	Effective	Highly effective	Not applicable	Comments
Presented or explained content clearly					
Used good examples to clarify points					
Varied explanations to respond to student questions or needs for clarification					
Emphasised important points					
Used graphics or visual aids or other enhancements to support presentation					
Used appropriate voice volume and inflection					
Presented information or led discussions with enthusiasm and interest					
Responded appropriately to student behaviours indicating boredom or confusion					
Summary					

Class interactions

The teacher:	Needs improvement	Effective	Highly effective	Not applicable	Comments
Encouraged student questions					
Asked questions to monitor student understanding					
Waited sufficient time for students to answer questions					
Provided opportunities for students to interact together to discover/discuss or practise content points					
Summary					

Teacher attitudes

The teacher:	Needs improvement	Effective	Highly effective	Not applicable	Comments
Showed enthusiasm for the content					
Showed respect for student questions and answers					
Summary					

Mastery of content

The teacher:	Needs improvement	Effective	Highly effective	Not applicable	Comments
Presented content at an appropriate level for the students					
Presented material relevant to the purpose of the course					
Demonstrated command of the subject matter					
Summary					

Course documents

The teacher:	Needs improvement	Effective	Highly effective	Not applicable	Comments
Provided appropriate handout materials to support lecture					
Provided additional supportive material to aid in student learning					
Summary					

Glossary

Here is a quick guide to some terms you will have come across within the book or may come across during your time as a teacher. These are not necessarily precise dictionary definitions but rather how they are used within the context of teaching and learning.

360 degree assessment
: An assessment method, often conducted anonymously, that is designed to provide feedback from multiple sources – for example, from self-assessment and peer assessment. The 360 degrees refers to a circle, suggesting that the person being evaluated or assessed is at the centre of the circle.

Action research
: This can be described as a continual process of planning, doing and then reviewing and reflecting to lead to another cycle of planning. It is often compared to Kolb's learning cycle but, generally, action research focuses on teams or processes rather than individuals in the process.

Active learning
: A learning process centred on the need to solve a real problem that involves action, reflection and personal development.

Andragogy
: Methods or techniques used to teach adults (as distinguished from techniques used to teach children, or 'pedagogy').

Blended learning
: Combining the best of face-to-face and elearning. Examples of blended learning include combinations of classroom instruction, online discussions, group activities and reflective journal tasks.

Case-Based Discussion (CBD)	A method of assessing clinical judgement, decision-making and application of knowledge. It involves a structured in-depth discussion between an experienced practitioner (the assessor) and the learner of a clinical event that the learner was intrinsically involved with.
Case-based learning	A clinical learning technique whereby patient data (in a de-identified or composite format) are presented as a problem-solving mechanism.
Case study	An example of a real-world situation. Case studies are used to demonstrate theoretical concepts in an applied setting.
Collaborative learning	Also known as cooperative learning. A process of getting two or more students to work together to achieve learning outcomes.
Competence	The ability to carry out a job or task.
Competency	A quality or characteristic of a person related to effective or superior performance. A competency is made up of many things such as knowledge, skills, attitudes, motives or traits.
Contact hours	The time spent in direct face-to-face contact with a teacher.
Curriculum	In its simplest form a curriculum is the range or set of courses that are offered by your establishment. It tends to be prescriptive, which means that students are aware of what they can study. For each course, there will be an underlying syllabus that describes the content of the course.
Deep learning approach	This involves linking new information to already known concepts, leading to understanding and long-term retention of information.
Didactic approach	Although 'didactic' literally means instructive, it also has connotations of an approach to teaching whereby the focus is on the presentation of information rather than the understanding of that information. In clinical teaching, it is sometimes used to differentiate 'classroom-based' activities from 'clinic-based' (or experiential) activities.

Distance learning	Education delivered to students who are not physically 'on site'.
Educational objectives	What the teacher aims to achieve.
eLearning	Learning using information and communication technology.
Experiential learning	Learning from direct experience. In clinical teaching, this would include learning from a clerkship, placement or internship in a healthcare practice setting.
Formative assessment	Assessment that informs the learner of their current progress and is not given a score or mark that counts towards their performance.
Inter-professional learning	Where learners from more than one profession learn together with the aim of also learning about and from each other in order to improve collaboration, foster multidisciplinary working and ultimately enhance the quality of patient care.
Learner-focused or learner-centred approach	An educational approach that focuses on the needs of the learner rather than the teacher or learning institution.
Learning aim	What is intended to be covered by the teacher in the course.
Learning management system (LMS)	A system designed to create a virtual learning environment in which one can use a variety of online instructional and assessment strategies.
Learning objective	Specific statements of learning intention.
Learning outcome	Clear statements of what the learner is expected to achieve when completing the course, and how they are expected to demonstrate that achievement.
Learning style	An approach or way of learning. It is thought that individuals have preferred ways of learning and that teaching strategies that match these styles can maximise student learning.

Mini-CEX	The Mini Clinical Evaluation Exercise assesses a practitioner 'one-to-one' in the context of their clinical environment. In this context, 'mini' refers to the fact that this is a shortened version of the original.
Mini-PAT	The Mini Peer Assessment Tool provides feedback to a learner from the perspective of co-workers who witness the learner's performance and practice. In this context, 'mini' refers to the fact that this is a shortened version of the original.
Multiple Choice Question (MCQ)	An MCQ is a form of assessment in which respondents must select the best possible answer (or answers) out of the choices from a list. Many different types of MCQs can be formed from a simple selection to a reasoning approach.
Notional hours	An estimate of the amount of time it will take for the learner to achieve the targeted level of competence. It consists of contact time with the lecturer and independent learning activities.
Objective Structured Clinical Examination (OSCE)	The OSCE assesses not only knowledge and attitudes but also communication and practical skills. Oriented around a station-based system, the focus of assessment changes with each station.
Ongoing assessment	This tracks student learning by performance on tasks that are part of the course. Ongoing assessment provides accumulated data for summative analysis.
Peer assessment or evaluation	An assessment or evaluation conducted by one's peers.
Philosophy of teaching	A formal written document of one's beliefs and attitudes towards teaching and learning.
Preceptor	An expert or specialist who gives practical experience and training to a student, particularly in the health professions.

Problem-based learning (PBL)	A learning approach whereby a group of students work together to solve problems and reflect on their experiences.
Professional socialisation	The process by which health professions students learn and internalise the roles, values, and expected behaviours of the intended profession.
Record of In-Training Assessment (RITA)	This is intended as an annual 'stop-check' on progress to ensure standards of training by assessing against a set of criteria. The RITA is supported by a portfolio of evidence detailing an individual's activities and learning.
Self-directed learning	Where an individual is personally responsible for achieving the required competencies, supported by the infrastructure of an accredited training centre.
Service learning	A teaching and learning method in which students learn by participating in and reflecting on activities that meet an identified need in the community.
SMART learning outcomes	Outcomes that are Specific, Measurable, Achievable, Realistic and delivered with a realistic Timeframe.
Social networking	A process of creating communities of people with similar interests. Examples include Facebook, MySpace and Twitter.
Subjective assessment	An assessment in which there may be more than one correct answer (or more than one way of expressing the correct answer).
Summative assessment	Assessment taken at the end of a period of learning in order to sum up achievement. A score is given that counts towards the student's final performance.
Surface learning approach	Memorising information and facts so that it leads to superficial retention of learning material that does not promote understanding or long-term retention of knowledge and information.

Teaching strategy	The combination of teaching and learning methods that are used to achieve desired educational outcomes.
Test-item analysis	An analysis that judges each item against pre-defined external criteria or against the remaining items in the assessment.
Viva voce; viva	An oral examination, usually to defend a thesis or dissertation.

Final thoughts

We hope you have enjoyed reading this quick guide to learning how to teach in the health professions. You will now be familiar with some key concepts, principles and theories involved in teaching and learning and will have some useful references and sources for further information if you wish to know more.

You will be aware of what is involved in developing course material and the common assessment techniques used in universities and in clinical practice.

You will also know that individuals have preferred learning styles, and that you can maximise learning through a mix of strategies and approaches which will suit all your students.

You may be ready to develop your own philosophy of teaching and, after your first teaching sessions, be able to evaluate your teaching, reflect on what went well, and develop ways to improve and enhance your practice.

The exercises, top tips and signposting to further reading and information resources will help you on your journey as a new teacher. We wish you all the best.

Suggestions for further reading

Adair J (1984). *The Skills of Leadership*. Aldershot: Gower.

Barnett R (2005). *Reshaping the University*. Buckingham: SRHE Open University Press.

Barnett R (2007). *A Will to Learn; Being a Student in an Age of Uncertainty*. Buckingham: SRHE Open University Press.

Barnett R, Coate K (2006). *Engaging the Curriculum in Higher Education*. Buckingham: SRHE Open University Press.

Biggs J, Tang C (2007). *Teaching for Quality Learning at University*, 3rd edn. Buckingham: SRHE Open University Press.

Bloxham S, Boyd P (2007). *Developing Effective Assessment in Higher Education*. Maidenhead: Open University Press.

Brockbank A, McGill I (2007). *Facilitating Reflective Learning in Higher Education*, 2nd edn. Buckingham: SRHE/Open University Press.

Brown S, Glasner A (1999). *Assessment Matters in Higher Education. Choosing and Using Diverse Approaches*. Buckingham: SRHE Open University Press.

Carr D (2000). *Professionalism and Ethics in Teaching*, London: RoutledgeFalmer.

Department for Business, Innovations and Skills (2009). *Higher Ambitions: The Future of Universities in a Knowledge Economy*. London: The Stationary Office.

Dewey J (1910). *How We Think.* Boston: D.C. Heath &Co. [(1994) New York: Prometheus].

Jarvis P (2006). *Towards a Comprehensive Theory of Human Learning,* London: Routledge-Falmer.

Light G, Cox R (2001). *Learning and Teaching in Higher Education: The Reflective Professional.* London: Paul Chapman Publishing.

Paechter C, Edwards R, Harrison R, Twining P (2001). *Learning Space and Identity.* London: Sage.

Ramsden P (2003). *Learning to Teach in Higher Education,* 2nd edn. London: Routledge-Falmer.

Schön D (1991). *The Reflective Practitioner: How Professionals Think in Action.* New York: Basic Books.

Tight M (2002). *Key Concepts in Adult Education and Training,* 2nd edn. London: RoutledgeFalmer.

Toohey S (1999). *Designing Courses in Higher Education.* Buckingham: SRHE Open University Press.

Wisker G, Clarke J, Exley K (2006). *One to One Teaching.* London: RoutledgeFalmer.

Index